YOUR PERSONAL NUTRITIONIST:

FIBER & FAT COUNTER

THE FACTS, THE FIGURES, THE BENEFITS—IT'S ALL IN THIS INVALUABLE GUIDE

- The sweet, satisfying food that is the most overlooked—and perhaps the best—source of dietary fiber
- Why fruit rolls and other kids' "fruit" treats should be avoided
- Why psyllium, the popular fiber supplement (and the active ingredient in those "natural" laxatives) may not be the best choice for you
- How to change your kids' favorite high-sugar cereal into a high-fiber dish . . . without them ever suspecting
- Which popular brand of hot dog bun turns out to be a great fiber choice
- What side dishes will change a zero-fiber, meat-based dinner into a heart-healthy meal
- Which snacks will satisfy your appetite and provide 3 to 4 grams of fiber while you munch (And check out those fabulous low or no-fat brands!)

YOUR PERSONAL NUTRITIONIST:

FIBER & FAT COUNTER

Ed Blonz, Ph.D.

A SIGNET BOOK

SIGNET

Published by the Penguin Group
Penguin Books USA Inc., 375 Hudson Street,
New York, New York 10014, U.S.A.
Penguin Books Ltd, 27 Wrights Lane, London W8 5TZ, England
Penguin Books Australia Ltd, Ringwood, Victoria, Australia
Penguin Books Canada Ltd, 10 Alcorn Avenue, Toronto, Ontario, Canada M4V 3B2
Penguin Books (N.Z.) Ltd, 182–190 Wairau Road, Auckland 10, New Zealand

Penguin Books Ltd, Registered Offices:
Harmondsworth, Middlesex, England

First published by Signet, an imprint of Dutton Signet,
a division of Penguin Books USA Inc.

First Printing, March, 1996
10 9 8 7 6 5 4 3 2 1

CONTENTS

CONTENTS

INTRODUCTION

Grandma Called It Roughage

Some people find the topic of fiber rather dry. That's appropriate, because that's how pure fiber tastes! But fiber's assets as a health promoter cannot be denied. You're about to learn what makes fiber so special. In addition, you've got your hands on a handy reference that lists the fiber content—along with the calories and fat—of almost 3,000 foods.

This booklet will help you boost the level of fiber in your diet. It will speed up your shopping trip by identifying foods that are high in fiber. Once you learn all that fiber has going for it, you'll be able to put this information to immediate use through a more fiber-conscious selection of ingredients and prepared foods.

What's So Special About Fiber?

About 90 percent of the time we've been on this planet, our diet has been high in fiber and low in fat. Only in the last two hundred years, following the Industrial Revolution, has our diet shifted toward more fat and less fiber.

Our palates were quick to embrace this change, but as health statistics suggest, our bodies haven't had the same success.

Population studies associate that earlier, fiber-rich way of eating with a lower incidence of heart disease and cancer, now the top two killer diseases in the U.S. In the countries of Africa and Asia, where the move to high fat never occurred, these diseases are almost nonexistent. Likewise, when individuals from a low-fat culture shift to the American way of eating, they begin to experience heart disease and cancer at the same rate that we do.

In addition to heart disease and cancer, a considerable body of research has accumulated linking an increased fiber intake (25 to 30 grams a day) with positive effects on diabetes, constipation, diarrhea, diverticulitis, hemorrhoids, and ulcerative colitis.

Today, just about every nutrition book and newsletter trumpets the praises of fiber without explaining what it is and what it does. So before you grab your next oat bran muffin, here's a look behind the labels.

All This and ZERO Calories, too!

Dietary fiber, or roughage, is a type of carbohydrate that's found only in plant products such as vegetables, nuts, fruits, and grains.

Fiber's imposing set of talents is made even more impressive when you consider that it doesn't contribute any calories, essential vitamins, or minerals to the body. In fact, it's not digested by the body at all! How can a substance we can't even digest be so healthful? The very fact that you cannot digest it is what turns out to be its greatest asset.

Why Fiber Can't Be Digested

The foods we eat are made up of a complex combination of nutrients and nonnutrient ingredients. In order for your body to absorb and use your food, it first has to take the food apart piece by piece. This *dis*-assembly line is your digestive system, a 26-foot-long muscular tube.

The "workers" along the digestive tract are enzymes, which are chemicals that can break apart the proteins, carbohydrates, or fats in food. Each of the dozen or so enzymes needed to digest a typical meal can perform only one action on one nutrient. For example, one enzyme specializes in splitting big proteins into smaller pieces, but a different enzyme is needed to complete the job.

Fiber is unique because the body completely lacks the enzymes it needs to take it apart. This means that instead of being absorbed like the other carbohydrates we eat, fiber becomes part of the bulk that travels through the small intestines into and through the large intestines, and eventually out of the body.

The word "fiber" doesn't refer to one substance. Rather, it stands for a variety of indigestible materials that are found in plant foods. As it travels through the body, each type of fiber acts according to how it's built. An important distinction is whether the fiber dissolves in water, so there are two main categories of dietary fiber: *insoluble* and *soluble,* and their health benefits differ.

Insoluble Fiber

The most familiar of the insoluble fibers is wheat bran, but it is also found in vegetables, fruits, and whole grains such as corn, rye, barley, and brown rice. Insoluble fiber increases the bulk and weight of the stool as well as the rate at which food travels through the digestive system. This can help your body ward off cancer. Population studies routinely find that the incidence of colon cancer goes down as the intake of insoluble fiber goes up. That's because fiber can effectively dilute or even grab on to potential cancer-causing substances and quickly usher them out of the body. That's some bodyguard!

Insoluble fiber also gets mixed with the bile salts, the digestive juice produced by the liver that helps with the absorption of dietary fats. Because the liver makes its bile salts from cholesterol, this binding action by insoluble fiber causes more cholesterol to leave the body.

Soluble Fiber

The most famous soluble fiber is probably oat bran, but this type of fiber is also found in rice bran, legumes (beans, lentils, and peas), fruits, and vegetables. Although these fibers dissolve in water, the body cannot absorb them because of their large size. Soluble fiber can't match the ability of insoluble fiber to add bulk, but it is more effective at lowering elevated blood cholesterol levels. It can, however, improve conditions connected with diabetes because it tends to slow the rate at which the body absorbs sugar. In addition, through a complex series of reactions, soluble fiber has a demonstrated ability to help lower blood cholesterol levels. Fruits and vegetables often contain both soluble and insoluble fibers. This is further proof of the wisdom of including them in your diet.

The bottom line: both soluble and insoluble fibers make major contributions to health and both should be included in your daily diet.

What's the Word on Oat Bran?

By now, oat bran has a war-weary media personality. After taking the fast track to food fame as a cholesterol-lowering food, oat bran experienced a precipitous drop in popularity following media stories that smeared its reputation. These reports were based on a journal study that found that oat bran was no better at lowering blood cholesterol than low-fiber wheat flour. Left out, however, was the fact that subjects in this particular study were young and middle-aged women with normal cholesterol levels. By contrast, most of the studies that established oat bran's cholesterol-lowering ability were performed on older men with elevated cholesterol levels.

The stage had been set, however, for this fall from grace. Oat bran had been overmarketed as a magic bullet that could turn virtually anything into cholesterol-busting health food. During its heyday, food manufacturers scrambled to add oat bran to everything under the sun. Nutritionists seemed to sit on their hands as all this was happening. They seemed grateful that people were finally interested in adding fiber to their diets—even if it meant recommending such bizarre creations as oat bran donuts.

If there's one thing we can learn from the oat-bran affair it's the need to appreciate the nature of scientific journalism. When a research report makes the transition from journal to headline news, the dropping of key details can greatly influence the public's perception. A journalist with science savvy needs to be somewhere in the loop to make sure everything is handled correctly. With oat bran, this didn't happen.

Oat bran was, and is, a good source of soluble fiber. Scientific studies continue to show that oat bran is a great addition to a healthy diet. The key dietary lesson to learn from the oat-bran affair is that there are no magic bullets in nutrition. The healthiness of a diet is measured by the foods we eat—not the fiber we add.

A Neglected Star: Dried Fruit

Dried fruit is a fabulous and often overlooked source of fiber. Figs and dates contain 9 grams of fiber per half-cup serving; prunes contain 7 grams per serving, and apricots and raisins contain 5 grams. By comparison, a slice of whole-wheat bread or a half cup of broccoli contain about 2 grams of dietary fiber.

In addition to its fiber content, dried fruit is also an excellent source of B vitamins and minerals. The pick of the group is the fig, also one of the richest nondairy sources of calcium. One serving of figs contains 144 milligrams of calcium, which on an ounce-by-ounce basis places them higher than milk. Figs are also a good source of iron, vitamin B-6, magnesium, and copper. Apricots are also a standout because one serving provides 25 percent of the U.S. Food and Drug Administration's Daily Value (DV) for iron and enough beta-carotene to satisfy almost 75 percent of the DV for vitamin A.

These high-fiber fruits are perfect as a nutritious snack—at home, in a child's lunch box, or stashed in a drawer for a workday nibble. They're also good chopped up in cottage cheese or yogurt, or in cereals or pancake mixes, where they can eliminate the need for added sugar. By rotating among the different fruits, you lend flavor and variety to the morning routine while adding nutritional value to the meal.

Be wary, however, of the fruit rolls and all other fabricated fruit doodads aimed at youngsters. These pseudo-fruits are packaged in wrappers covered with popular children's characters, such as Ghostbusters, Ninja Turtles, and Mario Brothers, as well as dinosaurs, clowns, and jet fighters. The makers want to cajole parents into choosing the products as a convenient way to add fruit to their children's diet and as an alternative to candy. But although these products boast that they are made with "real fruit," most primarily consist of a gummy fiberless sugar concoction that pales in comparison to the genuine article.

What About Fiber Supplements?

Many people take fiber supplements to relieve periodic constipation. Supplement use has grown as information on fiber's other benefits has spread—especially soluble fiber's cholesterol-lowering potential.

Psyllium, a popular fiber supplement, comes from the seeds of the plantago plant, a native to India and the Mediterranean. Used as a laxative in India for centuries, psyllium is also the main ingredient of over-the-counter laxatives in the U.S. On a weight basis, soluble fiber makes up 75 percent of the psyllium seed compared to oat bran's 8 percent soluble fiber. Studies have reported that adding psyllium, a soluble fiber, to the diet can help lower elevated blood cholesterol levels. Psyllium, however, offers little besides fiber. By contrast, oat bran is a good source of protein, magnesium, iron, zinc, thiamine, and phosphorus.

According to a recent report in the *American Journal of Clinical Nutrition* (AJCN), *when* you take the psyllium—with or between meals—is an important consideration. In the AJCN study, 18 men and women with elevated cholesterol levels were given psyllium either with a meal or one and a half hours before the meal. It was only when the psyllium was taken with the meal that the cholesterol-lowering effect was observed.

Don't Add Too Much Too Fast

Although fiber is good for you, you don't want to add too much of it too fast. The result could be an overstimulated digestive system. When you rapidly increase the level in your diet—a particular problem with supplements—there is a greater chance of short-term side effects such as bloating, cramps, diarrhea, and gas. In addition, an overload of fiber can interfere with the absorption of nutrients. This can be a particular problem with supplements like psyllium. Medications may also be affected, so if you're taking any, talk to your health professional before adding any fiber supplements to your diet.

A good strategy is to slowly integrate the high-fiber foods into your daily routine until you arrive at a comfortable level. Portion control may be needed with children, as they may quickly develop a taste for sweet high-fiber dried apricots, figs, prunes, and raisins.

Food Labels Are More Informative

Good news: the Food and Drug Administration has cleared up the language on food labels. If a product label says either **"contains fiber"** or **"good source of fiber,"** there must be between 2.5 and 4.9 grams of fiber per serving. If a label says **"high"** in fiber or **"rich"** in fiber, that means there will be at least 5 grams per serving.

Figuring Out Your Fiber Strategy

At present, the typical American diet contains about 12 to 15 grams of dietary fiber per day. Most authorities recommend twice this amount, up to at least 25 to 30 grams per day. **An adequate fiber intake is an essential part of a healthy diet.**

There are many ways to give your diet the fiber boost it needs. The key is being able to make more fiber-conscious food selections. That comes from knowing where the fiber is—and where it isn't. With the information contained in these pages, you're on your way!

Checking to see how your current diet stacks up is a good first step. By skimming through this booklet you'll be able to get a good idea where your current diet stands on the fiber scale. Then, take a look at the food categories you normally include in your daily diet and which choices might represent better alternatives.

Sprucing up a fiber-poor diet is not that difficult. Here are some easy substitutions to help you reach your goal.

Instead of:	Try:	Fiber Gain
Buttermilk pancakes	Buckwheat pancakes	+ 1 g
White bread	Whole grain bread	+ 2 g
Flour crackers	Whole wheat or rye crackers	+ 2 g
White rice	Brown rice	+ 2 g

French fries	Side salad	+ 3 g
Potato chips	High-fiber pretzels or chips	+ 3 g
Potato chips	Banana	+ 4 g
Regular hamburger bun	High-fiber bun	+ 4 g
Flour pasta	Whole-grain pasta	+ 5 g
Chicken noodle soup	Split pea soup	+ 6 g
Sauce or gravy	with 2 tablespoons oat bran	+ 6 g
White flour	Whole wheat flour	+ 7 g
Flour tortillas	Whole wheat tortillas	+ 8 g
Chili without beans	Chili with beans	+ 10 g
Cereal	Cereal with ½ cup dry blueberries	+ 10 g
Second helping of meat	Serving of carrot-raisin salad	+ 16 g
Fruit rollup	Dried figs or apricots	+ 10–18 g
Low-fiber cereals	Bran-based cereals	+ 5–25 g

The Tables Ahead

The tables in this pamphlet are specifically designed to let you see which types of foods have the highest levels of dietary fiber. It will also let you compare fiber content among similar foods. And to help you make more healthful food choices, the pamphlet also lists the amount of fat and calories in each portion. A check mark (✓) next to an entry means that that food is a good source of fiber, providing at least 5 grams per serving.

The listings are separated into convenient food categories. Whenever possible, similar foods have been listed in comparable portion sizes. As you look through the listings, you'll see that there may be variations in fiber content—even among similar types of foods. This can be due to the fact that different manufacturers rely on different raw materials to make their product.

The data in these tables come from a number of sources, including product labels, manufacturers' information, the United States Dept. of Agriculture (Agricultural Handbooks No. 8), the Canadian Nutrition Foundation, and the Produce Marketing Association.

BEVERAGES

You won't find many high-fiber foods in the beverage category. Milk, although a nutritious food, has no fiber, and sodas, coffee, and alcoholic beverages are little more than flavored water.

Fiber can be found, however, in juices made from fresh vegetables, such as carrots and tomatoes, and fruit such as prunes, passion fruit, and oranges when they are made fresh with the pulp included. There are some cocoa powders that contain fiber-based thickeners, which add smoothness to the drink.

ITEM NAME	PORTION	CAL	FAT	FIBER
Beef Broth & Tomato Juice				
Beverage	1 cup	88	0.0	1.6
Beer, Light	1 cup	66	0.0	0.0
Beer, Regular (5% Alcohol)	1 cup	105	0.0	1.2
Carnation Instant Breakfast	1 item	130	0.0	0.0
Cocoa Mix, Powdered, Fortified	1 serv.	120	3.0	0.7
Cocoa Mix, Chocolate Flavor,				
Prepared - Ovaltine	1 cup	227	8.8	0.2
Cocoa, Prepared with Milk - Home				
Recipe	1 cup	218	9.1	3.0
Coffee (unflavored)	—	—	—	0.0
Coffee (flavored)				
Instant Cappuccino - Nescafe	1 env.	110	2.0	0.5
Swiss Mocha - Hills Brothers	1⅓ tbps.	45	2.0	0.5
Egg Nog - Lucerne	1 cup	340	18.0	0.0
Fruit Punch, Powder/Water	1 cup	97	0.0	0.2
Liqueurs	—	—	—	0.0
Meal Replacement - Slimfast,				
Vanilla, w/Skim Milk	1 cup	190	1.0	2.0
Meal replacement, Sweet				
Success - Nestle	1 cup	160	2.4	4.8
Milk (see DAIRY)				
Orange Drink, Vitamin,				
Powder/Water	1 cup	118	0.0	0.2
Sodas, Assorted Flavors,				
Diet & Regular, Carbonated	—	—	—	0
Soy Milk, Fluid	1 cup	79	4.6	3.1
Soy Moo (Imitation Milk),				
Fat Free - Health Valley	1 cup	110	0.0	1.0
Squeezit 100 Flavored Drink -				
Betty Crocker	1 btle.	110	0.0	0.0
Tea	—	—	—	0.0
Wine, Red, White or Rose	—	—	—	0.0
Wine Coolers	1 cup	117	1.4	0.1

ITEM NAME	PORTION	CAL	FAT	FIBER

FRUIT & VEGETABLE JUICES

ITEM NAME	PORTION	CAL	FAT	FIBER
Apple Cider	1 cup	124	0.3	0.2
Apple Juice, Canned or Bottled	1 cup	116	0.3	0.5
Apricot Nectar, Canned	1 cup	141	0.2	1.5
✔ Carrot Juice, Canned	1 cup	98	0.4	5.9
Cranberry Grape Juice, Bottled	1 cup	137	0.2	0.1
Grapefuit Juice, Fresh	1 cup	96	0.2	0.5
Lemon Juice, Fresh	1 cup	61	0.0	0.7
Lemonade, Aspartame, Sweet, Powder/Water	1 cup	5	0.0	0.4
Lemonade, Frozen Concentrate, Diluted	1 cup	105	0.0	0.6
Limeade, Frozen Concentrate, Diluted	1 cup	100	0.0	0.5
Orange Grapefruit Juice, Canned	1 cup	106	0.2	0.5
Orange Juice, Fresh	1 cup	111	0.5	2.0
Orange Juice, Frozen Concentrate, Diluted	1 cup	109	0.1	0.8
Papaya Nectar	1 cup	143	0.4	1.2
Passion Fruit Juice, Purple	1 cup	126	0.1	3.4
Passion Fruit Juice, Yellow	1 cup	148	0.4	1.3
Peach Nectar, Canned	1 cup	134	.01	0.4
Pineapple Grapefruit Juice, Canned	1 cup	118	0.3	0.3
Pineapple Juice Frozen Concentrate	1 cup	130	0.1	0.3
Pineapple Orange Juice, Vitamin C, Canned	1 cup	125	0.0	0.4
Prune Juice, Canned & Bottled	1 cup	182	0.1	2.6
Tangerine Juice				
Fresh	1 cup	106	0.5	0.8
Frozen Concentrate	1 cup	110	0.3	0.5
Tomato & Clam Juice, Clamato - Motts	1 cup	111	0.2	1.5
Tomato Juice				
Campbell's	1 cup	50	0.0	1.0
Low Sodium	1 cup	42	0.1	2.8
Vegetable Juice				
Canned	1 cup	46	0.2	2.7
Snap-E-Tom	1 cup	46	0.0	1.9
V8, Regular - Campbell's	1 cup	49	0.0	2.4
V8, Spice Hot - Campbell's	1 cup	49	0.0	1.4

BREADS & BREADSTUFFS

Breads and breadstuffs are often loaded with fiber. But it all depends on whether the item is made from fiber-rich whole grain flour or a "white flour" in which the fiber has been removed. Although foods made with whole grain flours tend to be darker in color, you can't rely on color as your only guide. Some brown-colored breads owe their darker color to added food coloring, and many food companies add fiber to the dough of their "white" breads to improve the nutritional value. Use this list to spot your best high-fiber choices.

ITEM NAME	PORTION	CAL	FAT	FIBER
BAGELS				
Cinnamon Raisin - Sara Lee	1 bagel	290	1.0	4.0
Cinnamon Raisin - Thomas'	1 bagel	170	2.0	3.0
Egg, Frozen - Lenders	1 bagel	160	1.0	1.0
Garlic - Noah's	1 bagel	320	1.0	2.4
New York Caraway Rye - Noah's	1 bagel	310	2.0	3.0
Onion, Frozen - Lenders	1 bagel	160	1.0	2.0
Plain, Frozen - Lenders	1 bagel	160	1.0	1.0
Plain - Noah's	1 bagel	320	1.0	2.4
Poppy Seed - Noah's	1 bagel	320	1.0	2.4
BISCUITS				
Baking Powder, 1869 - Pillsbury	1 biscuit	100	5.0	0.3
Biscotti, Almond	1 biscuit	168	9.0	2.0
Butter/Buttermilk or Country - Pillsbury	1 biscuit	50	1.0	0.2
Butter Tastin - Big Country	1 biscuit	100	4.0	0.4
Flaky, Hungry Jack - Pillsbury	1 biscuit	80	4.0	0.3
Gold Medal, Mix	1 biscuit	90	4.0	0.4
Good N Buttery, Fluffy	1 biscuit	90	5.0	0.4
Heat N Eat, Big Premium - Pillsbury	1 biscuit	140	8.0	2.7
Southern, Big Country - Pillsbury	1 biscuit	100	4.0	0.4
BREADS				
Apple/Cinnamon - Quick Bread Mix	1 serv.	140	1.0	0.3
Banana - Quick Bread Mix	1 serv.	120	1.0	0.3
Blueberry - Quick Bread Mix	1 serv.	130	1.0	0.3
Breadstick				
Italian - Barbara's	1 item	35	1.0	1.0
Onion - Keebler	1 item	15	0.0	0.1
Plain - Colombo	1 item	40	0.0	1.3

ITEM NAME	PORTION	CAL	FAT	FIBER
Sesame - Keebler	1 item	15	1.0	0.1
Soft - Pillsbury	1 item	100	2.0	1.0
Sourdough - Bread Du Jour	1 biscuit	130	1.0	1.0
Bread Crumbs				
Dry, Grated	1 cup	390	5.0	3.7
Dry, Plain - Toscana	1 cup	440	4.0	2.0
Dry, Seasoned - Colombo	1 cup	440	4.0	2.0
Buttermilk, Hearty - Home Pride	1 slice	100	2.0	0.8
Carrot Elfin Loaves - Keebler	1 item	210	10.0	0.8
Cinnamon Raisin - Wonder	1 slice	70	1.0	0.8
Cornbread - Ballard	1 serv.	120	2.0	0.6
Cornbread Twists - Pillsbury	1 item	70	4.0	0.4
✔ Cranberry Elfin Loaves - Keebler	1 item	160	6.0	5.0
Crisp, Whole Grain - Wasa	1 slice	22	0.0	0.5
Date - Quick Bread Mix	1 serv.	140	1.0	0.3
Egg (Challah)	1 slice	206	8.0	1.0
Fat Free, Buttermilk - Orowheat	1 slice	40	0.0	2.0
Foccacia - Dicarlo's	1/8 slice	130	2.0	1.0
French				
Bread Du Jour (3" slices)	1 slice	130	1.0	1.0
Loaf, Crusty - Pillsbury	1 slice	60	1.0	0.8
Parisian - Dicarlo's	1 slice	35	1.0	0.6
Wonder Light	1 slice	40	1.0	2.5
Gingerbread - Pillsbury	1 serv.	180	5.0	0.4
Granola - Wonder	1 slice	50	1.0	1.0
Honey Bran, Light - Wonder	1 slice	40	<1.0	3.0
Italian				
Mrs. Wrights	1 slice	90	1.0	1.0
Wonder Light	1 slice	40	1.0	2.5
Melba Toast, Plain or Wheat	1 slice	16	0.0	0.3
Multi Grain (7 Grain), Hearty - Home Pride	1 slice	100	2.0	2.0
Nine Grain - Wonder Light	1 slice	40	1.0	3.0
Nut - Quick Bread Mix	1 serv.	150	3.0	0.1
Oat, Fat Free - Orowheat	1 slice	40	0.0	2.5
Oat Bran - Monterey	1 slice	99	1.0	3.3
✔ Oat Bran Elfin Loaves, Fiber - Keebler	1 item	170	6.0	5.0
Oatmeal	1 slice	65	1.0	0.5
Pepperidge Farm	1 slice	90	1.0	1.0
Wonder Light	1 slice	45	1.0	2.0
Oatmeal & Bran - Oatmeal Goodness	1 slice	90	2.0	1.0
Oatmeal/Raisin - Quick Bread Mix	1 serv.	140	2.0	0.3
Oats & Cracked Wheat, Hearty Honey - Home Pride	1 slice	100	2.0	2.0
Pita, White - Mr. Pita	1 pita	210	1.0	3.0

ITEM NAME	PORTION	CAL	FAT	FIBER
Pita, Whole Wheat - Mr. Pita	1 pita	220	2.0	4.0
Pumpernickel - Beefsteak	1 slice	70	1.0	1.0
Raisin Cinnamon Swirl - Sun Maid	1 slice	80	2.0	1.0
Sourdough				
Wonder	1 slice	90	1.0	0.8
Wonder Light	1 slice	40	1.0	2.5
Sourdough Baguette - Semifreddi's	1 slice	144	0.0	1.0
Taco Shell, Super - Old El Paso	1 item	100	6.0	1.5
Texas Toast - Wonder	1 slice	100	1.0	1.0
Tortilla, Corn - Mission	1 item	80	1.0	1.0
Tortilla, Flour				
✔ Fat Free - La Tortilla Factory	1 item	60	0.0	6.0
Low Fat - Wonder	1 item	110	2.0	1.0
Large - Senorita's	1 item	150	4.0	1.0
✔ Tortilla, Whole Wheat, Fat Free -				
La Tortilla Factory	1 item	60	0.0	9.0
Tortilla, Whole Wheat - Trader Joe's	1 item	140	5.0	3.0
Vienna - Wonder	1 slice	70	1.0	0.8
Rye Breads				
Fat Free - Orowheat	1 slice	50	0.0	2.5
Hearty Deli - Home Pride	1 slice	140	2.0	3.0
Light - Beefsteak	1 slice	35	1.0	2.5
Odessa-Semifreddi's	1 slice	134	0.0	1.0
Wonder	1 slice	70	1.0	1.0
Wonder Light	1 slice	35	1.0	2.5
White Wheat Breads				
Grain - Home Pride	1 slice	60	1.0	2.0
Hearty White - Beefsteak	1 slice	70	1.0	1.0
Home Pride	1 slice	70	1.0	1.0
Wonder	1 slice	70	1.0	0.8
"Wonder Kid" - Wonder	1 slice	60	1.0	2.0
Wonder Light	1 slice	40	1.0	2.5
Whole Grain Wheat Breads				
100% Stoneground - Home Pride	1 slice	90	2.0	3.0
100% Whole Grain - Wonder	1 slice	70	1.0	2.0
100% Whole Grain, Soft - Wonder	1 slice	55	1.0	1.0
Fat Free - Orowheat	1 slice	40	0.0	3.0
Firm, Enriched	1 slice	61	1.0	2.8
Other Wheat Breads				
Austrian - Bread Du Jour	1 slice	130	2.0	2.0
Cracked Wheat - Wonder	1 slice	70	1.0	1.0
Hearty Wheat - Home Pride	1 slice	100	2.0	0.8

ITEM NAME	PORTION	CAL	FAT	FIBER
Honey Wheat - Home Pride	1 slice	70	1.0	1.0
Light, Home Pride	1 slice	37	1.0	2.0
Old Fashioned - Orowheat	1 slice	70	1.0	0.4
Pipin' Hot, Loaf - Pillsbury	1 slice	70	2.0	0.7
Soft - Beefsteak	1 slice	70	1.0	0.8
Whole Wheat Blend, Light - Home Pride	1 slice	37	1.0	2.0
Wonder Light	1 slice	40	<1.0	2.5

CRACKERS

ITEM NAME	PORTION	CAL	FAT	FIBER
7 Grain Vegetable - Health Valley	1 oz.	110	4.0	3.8
Amaranth Graham, Fat Free - Health Valley	8 items	100	0.0	3.0
American Cheese/Wheat - Keebler	2 items	140	8.0	0.2
Barge Pilot Biscuits	1/3 cup	117	2.0	1.0
Bran Thins, Toasted - Nabisco	2 serv.	120	6.0	2.0
Butter Flavor, Original - Flutters	1 serv.	100	4.0	0.2
Cheddar Snacks - Ralston	18 items	130	5.0	1.8
Cheese, Cheeze-It				
Hot & Spicy - Sunshine	26 items	160	8.0	1.0
Reduced Fat - Sunshine	30 pieces	140	5.0	0.8
Regular - Sunshine	27 items	160	8.0	0.8
White Cheddar - Sunshine	26 items	160	9.0	0.5
Cheese & Chives - Ralston	18 items	130	5	1.8
Cheese Flavor, Organic - Health Valley	10 pieces	100	0.0	4.0
Club, Low Sodium - Keebler	2 serv.	120	6.0	0.6
Cracked Wheat - American Classic	2 serv.	140	8.0	1.6
Crispbread, Light Rye - Wasa	3 slices	75	0.0	3.0
Crispy Cheese - Cheddar Wedges	2 serv.	140	6.0	0.2
Dairy Butter - American Classic	2 serv.	140	6.0	0.2
Fire Crackers, All Varieties - Health Valley	12 pieces	100	0.0	4.0
Goldfish, Cheese - Pepperidge Farm	1 serv.	120	4.0	1.0
Graham, Chocolate Flavored - Nabisco	8 items	120	3.0	1.0
Graham, Cinnamon				
Honey Maid - Nabisco	10 items	140	3.0	1.0
Snackwell Fat Free - Nabisco	20 items	110	0.0	1.0
Graham, Fudge Dipped - Keebler	3 items	140	7.0	0.8
Graham, Honey,				
Fiber - Keebler	4 items	120	1.0	0.4
Health Valley	1 oz.	130	5.0	3.5
Keebler	4 items	140	4.0	0.8

ITEM NAME	PORTION	CAL	FAT	FIBER
Sunshine	2 items	120	4.0	1.0
Honey Maid - Nabisco	8 items	120	3.0	1.0
Graham Oat Bran - Health Valley	8 items	100	0.0	3.0
Harvest Crisps, - Nabisco	2 items	20	1.0	0.4
Herb, Organic - Health Valley	10 pieces	100	0.0	4.0
Herb, Stoned Wheat - Health Valley	1 oz.	110	4.0	3.8
Matzo Meal - Manischewitz	¼ cup	129	<1.0	1.0
Matzos - Manischewitz	1 serv.	115	2.0	0.8
Matzos, Daily Thin Tea - Manischewitz	1 piece	103	<1.0	0.7
Melba Snacks, Garlic/Onion - Old London	10 pieces	120	3.0	4.0
Melba Snacks, Sesame - Old London	10 pieces	120	6.0	2.0
Melba Toast				
Sesame - Devonsheer	6 pieces	10	2.0	2.0
Wheat - Devonsheer	6 pieces	10	0.0	1.8
Munchems, Original - Keebler	2 serv.	140	6.0	3.0
Oat Thins, Toasted - Nabisco	18 items	140	6.0	2.0
Onion, Organic - Health Valley	10 pieces	100	0.0	4.0
Oyster - Keebler	3 items	120	3.0	0.6
Peanut Butter/Cheese - Keebler	2 items	140	6.0	0.4
Pizza, Garlic/Herb & Cheese, Italiano - Health Valley	12 pieces	100	0.0	4.0
Rich & Crisp - Ralston	9 items	140	6.0	1.0
Ritz	9 items	162	9.0	1.0
Ry Krisp				
Natural - Ralston	13 items	98	0.0	4.0
✔ Seasoned - Ralston	13 items	108	3.0	5.2
Rye Snack, Toasted - Keebler	9 items	135	9.0	0.9
Rye Snacks - Ralston	15 items	131	6.0	4.5
Saltines				
Multigrain - Nabisco	10 items	120	3.0	1.0
Premium, No Fat - Nabisco	6 items	100	0.0	2.0
Zesta - Keebler	10 items	125	5.0	1.0
Sandwich, Crackers				
Cheese & Peanut Butter - Keebler	1 pkg.	190	9.0	0.8
Club & Cheddar - Keebler	1 pkg.	190	11.0	0.5
Toast & Peanut Butter - Keebler	1 pkg.	190	9.0	1.0
Sesame - American Heritage	9 items	160	9.0	1.0
Sesame & Wheat - Ralston	15 items	130	6.0	3.0
Snackers - Ralston	8 items	140	6.0	0.8
Sun Toasted Wheats - Keebler	2 items	14	1.0	0.6
Vegetable, Organic - Health Valley	10 pieces	100	0.0	4.0

ITEM NAME	PORTION	CAL	FAT	FIBER
Vegetable Thins - Nabisco	14 items	160	9.0	1.0
Wheat				
Keebler Harvest Wheats	2 items	30	2.0	1.4
Organic - Health Valley	10 pieces	100	0.0	4.0
Snackwell Fat Free - Nabisco	10 items	120	0.0	2.0
Wheat Thins - Nabisco	16 items	144	6.0	1.6
Wheat Thins, Multigrain - Nabisco	17 items	130	4.0	2.0
Wheatables, Ranch - Keebler	2 serv.	140	6.0	1.4
Wheatables, White Cheddar - Keebler	2 serv.	140	8.0	0.6
Wheatsworth Stone Ground - Nabisco	9 items	144	6.0	1.8
Wheetines - Barbara's	2 squares	120	2.0	0.0
Wheat & Bran - American Heritage	9 items	140	7.0	2.0
Wheat Snacks, Toasted - Keebler	9 items	135	9.0	0.9
Whole Wheat				
Fat Free, All Varieties - Health Valley	10 items	100	0.0	4.0
✔ Low Sodium	4 serv.	120	0	11.2
Triscuits - Nabisco	7 items	140	5.0	4.0
Wheat & Bran, Triscuits - Nabisco	7 items	140	5.0	4.0
Wholegrain Wheat - Keebler	8 items	120	4.0	1.6
Zwieback - Nabisco	3 items	105	3.0	1.0

MUFFINS

ITEM NAME	PORTION	CAL	FAT	FIBER
Apple Cin, Mix, RobinHood/Gold Medal	1 muffin	130	4.0	0.0
Australian Toaster Biscuit, Cornbread - Orowheat	1 muffin	200	3.0	2.0
Australian Toaster Biscuit, Plain - Orowheat	1 muffin	180	5.0	0.9
Banana, Fat Free - Health Valley	1 muffin	130	1.0	4.5
Banana Nut, Frozen - Weight Watchers	1 muffin	190	5.0	3.0
Banana Nut Mini - Hostess	1 muffin	52	3.0	0.2
Berry - Creamy Deluxe	1 muffin	100	3.0	0.4
Blueberry				
✔ Fat Free, Twin - Health Valley	1 muffin	140	1.0	5.0
Free & Light - Sara Lee	1 muffin	120	0.0	0.9
Blueberry Mini - Hostess	1 muffin	48	3.0	0.2
Blueberry Oat Bran - Health Valley	1 muffin	140	4.0	4.7
Bran - Home Recipe	1 muffin	112	5.0	2.5
Chocolate Chip Mini - Hostess	1 muffin	52	3.0	0.2
Cinnaminis, Original - Hostess	1 muffin	60	3.0	0.4

ITEM NAME	PORTION	CAL	FAT	FIBER
Corn - Home Recipe	1 muffin	125	4.0	1.0
✔ Crumpet	1 item	60	0.0	5.0
English				
Blueberry, Gourmet - Sara Lee	1 muffin	250	2.0	3.0
Health Nut Raisin	1 muffin	180	4.0	3.0
Oat Bran - Thomas	1 muffin	120	1.0	2.0
Oat Nut Bran - Orowheat	1 muffin	160	3.0	2.0
Raisin Rounds - Wonder	1 muffin	150	2.0	2.0
Regular - Wonder	1 muffin	120	1.0	1.0
Sourdough - Thomas'	1 muffin	120	1.0	1.0
✔ Fancy Fruit, Almond Date -				
Health Valley	1 muffin	140	1.0	8.2
Honey Bran, Mix -				
Robin Hood/Gold Medal	1 muffin	140	4.0	1.7
Oat, Mix - Robin Hood/Gold				
Medal	1 muffin	130	4.0	1.6
Oat Bran				
Hostess	1 muffin	160	8.0	0.8
Mix - Creamy Deluxe	1 muffin	170	7.0	2.0
✔ Raisin Oat Bran - Health Valley	1 muffin	140	3.0	5.2
✔ Raisin Spice, Fat Free -				
Health Valley	1 muffin	130	1.0	5.1
Soy	1 muffin	119	4.0	0.8

ROLLS & BUNS

ITEM NAME	PORTION	CAL	FAT	FIBER
Brown & Serve - Enriched	1 roll	85	2.0	1.0
Brown 'N Serve, Asst.-Wonder	1 roll	70	1.0	0.5
Cinnamon, 2 Pack - Pepperidge	1 oz.	124	6.0	0.5
Cloverleaf - Home Recipe	1 roll	120	3.0	1.3
Cracked Wheat, Bavarian -				
Bread Du Jour	1 roll	90	1.0	1.0
Croissant - Sara Lee	1 item	109	6.0	0.6
Dinner				
Butterflake - Pillsbury	1 roll	140	5.0	0.9
Crescent - Pillsbury	1 roll	100	6.0	0.6
✔ Tea, White - Wonder	1 roll	80	1.0	5.0
Wheat - Home Pride	1 roll	160	4.0	2.0
White - Home Pride	1 roll	65	2.0	0.5
White - Wonder Light	1 roll	60	1.0	4.0
French - Dicarlo's	1 slice	70	1.0	0.8
Hamburger				
Home Pride	1 bun	130	2.0	2.0
Wheat - Wonder	1 bun	170	3.0	1.0
Wonder	1 bun	110	2.0	0.8
✔ Wonder Light	1 bun	80	2.0	5.0

ITEM NAME	PORTION	CAL	FAT	FIBER
Hot Dog				
Home Pride	1 bun	130	2.0	2.0
Wonder	1 bun	110	2.0	0.8
✔ Wonder Light	1 bun	80	2.0	5.0
Italian, Crusty - Bread Du Jour	1 roll	80	1.0	0.8
Kaiser - Kilpatrick's	1 roll	180	3.0	1.0
Potato - Home Pride	1 roll	130	2.0	2.0
Rye - Bread Du Jour	1 roll	90	2.0	1.0
Sandwich, Wheat - Home Pride	1 roll	160	2.0	2.0
Sourdough - Bread Du Jour	1 roll	140	2.0	2.0
Sourdough, Extra - Dicarlo's	1 slice	100	1.0	1.0
Submarine/Hoagie, Enriched	1 roll	390	4.0	3.8
Whole Wheat, Homemade	1 roll	90	1.0	1.8

STUFFING

ITEM NAME	PORTION	CAL	FAT	FIBER
Chicken Flavor, Stove Top -				
General Foods	1 cup	220	3.0	2.0
Classic Chicken - Pepperidge	1 cup	220	2.0	0.2
Cornbread				
Orowheat	1 cup	330	3.0	1.5
Pepperidge	1 cup	226	3.0	2.7
Stove Top - General Foods	1 cup	220	2.0	2.6
Country Style - Pepperidge	1 cup	186	2.0	2.7
French Bread - Parisian	1 cup	160	1.0	2.0
Herb Butter & Wild Rice,				
Dry - Golden Grain	1 cup	300	3.0	3.0
Herb Seasoned - Pepperidge	1 cup	227	2.0	4.0
Pork, Stove Top - General				
Foods	1 cup	220	2.0	2.6
San Francisco Style Sour Dough,				
Dry Mix - Stove Top	1 cup	220	2.0	2.0
Seasoned - Orowheat	1 cup	110	1.0	2.0
Seasoned - Wonder	1 cup	60	1.0	0.8
Traditional - Butterball	1 cup	195	2.0	3.0
Turkey, Stove Top -				
General Foods	1 cup	220	2.0	2.0

OTHER

ITEM NAME	PORTION	CAL	FAT	FIBER
Capati	1 oz.	85	2.0	0.2
Croutons	1 cup	151	2.0	0.8
Croutons, Seasoned - Pepperidge	1 oz.	140	6.0	1.3
Pakoda	1 oz.	89	4.0	0.1
Papadam	1 oz.	146	9.0	0.1
Phyllo Dough - Athens Foods	1/8 pkg.	180	1.0	1.0

ITEM NAME	PORTION	CAL	FAT	FIBER
Pie Crust, Ready-made 9-Inch - Pillsbury	⅛ pkg.	110	7.0	0.0
Puff Pastry, Frozen - Pepperidge	⅙ sheet	200	11.0	3.0

BREAKFAST FOODS

High-fiber cereals are a great way to start the day, but they're also good food anytime you need a quick bite. In addition to their fiber content, they're a ready source of complex carbohydrates, vitamins, and minerals. But as anyone who's walked down a cereal aisle can tell you, they come in a wide variety of sizes, shapes, and colors. The variation also extends to their nutritional assets—and that means fiber. Check out the following list for the best sources. You'll find that the bran-based cereals provide a reliable fiber source, with a cup of an all-bran type cereal packing as much as 20 to 30 grams of fiber per cup. Cereals, however, can be made from a wide variety of grains—and different parts of the grain—ranging from fiber-rich whole grains to fiber-poor flours. To help provide a level playing ground, we've listed most items in one-cup servings, making exceptions for the dense, filling all-bran and granola type cereals. As you make your selections, be sure to check the label on the box as cereals vary *greatly* in the amount of fat and sugar per serving.

One special note for parents: children often get overly attached to sweet cereals that offer little in the way of nutritional value. Fiber-up their breakfast by mixing bran or bran-based cereal with their favorite morning cereal.

ITEM NAME	PORTION	CAL	FAT	FIBER
CEREALS				
Bran Cereals				
100% Organic Bran/Raisin - Health Valley	1 cup	160	0.0	4.9
✔ 100% Bran - Nabisco	½ cup	120	0.8	12.0
✔ 40% Bran Flakes - Kellogg's	1 cup	127	0.7	7.6
✔ 40% Bran Flakes - Post	1 cup	152	0.8	9.2
✔ All Bran - Kellogg's	½ cup	80	1.0	10.0
✔ All Bran with Extra Fiber - Kellogg's	⅓ cup	50	1.0	15.0
✔ Bran, Unprocessed - Quaker	5 tbsp.	30	0.0	8.0
✔ Bran Buds - Kellogg's	1 cup	210	3.0	11.0
✔ Bran Flakes - Post	1 cup	135	0.8	9.0
✔ Bran Flakes - Ralston	1 cup	159	0.7	6.0
Bran Flakes & Fruit	1 cup	179	0.7	4.6
✔ Common Sense Oat Bran - Kellogg's	1 cup	147	1.3	5.3
Common Sense Oat Bran/Raisins - Kellogg's	1 cup	160	2.0	4.8
✔ Complete Bran Flakes - Kellogg's	1 cup	133	0.7	6.7

ITEM NAME	PORTION	CAL	FAT	FIBER
✔ Corn Bran - Quaker	1 cup	120	1.3	6.7
✔ Cracklin Oat Bran - Kellogg's	1 cup	306	10.6	8.0
✔ Crunchy Bran - Quaker	1 cup	120	1.3	6.7
Frosted Bran - Kellogg's	1 cup	133	0.0	4.0
Fruitful Bran - Kellogg's	1 cup	136	0.8	4.8
✔ Harvest Crunch, Raisins & Bran	1 cup	442	20.9	8.3
Honey Bran	1 cup	119	1.0	3.9
✔ Honey Bran Crunchies	1 cup	184	1.0	6.6
✔ Mueslix Bran	1 cup	312	3.7	13.6
✔ Oat Bran - Quaker	1 cup	168	2.4	5.6
Organic Oat Bran Flakes - Health Valley	1 cup	133	0.0	5.3
Organic Oat Bran O's - Health Valley	1 cup	146	0.0	4.0
Raisin Bran				
✔ Kellogg's	1 cup	170	1.0	7.0
✔ Post	1 cup	190	1.0	8.0
✔ Ralston	1 cup	178	0.3	7.1
✔ Raisin Nut Bran - General Mills	1 cup	210	4.5	5.0
✔ Ripple Crisp Honey Bran - General Mills	1 cup	152	0.8	5.0
✔ Total Raisin Bran - General Mills	1 cup	180	1.0	5.0
✔ Wheat Bran - Kretschmer Toasted	4 tbsp.	30	1.0	7.0

Corn Cereals

ITEM NAME	PORTION	CAL	FAT	FIBER
Chex, Corn - Ralston	1 cup	88	0.0	1.0
Corn Flakes				
Kellogg's	1 cup	110	0.0	1.0
✔ Organic Blue Corn - Health Valley	1 cup	120	0.0	5.3
Ralston	1 cup	98	0.1	1.1
Corn Pops	1 cup	108	0.1	0.1
Corn, Shredded, Added Sugar	1 cup	95	0.0	1.5
Country Corn Flakes - General Mills	1 cup	120	0.5	0.5
Honey Nut Corn Flakes	1 cup	149	2.0	0.9
Lites, Puffed Corn - Health Valley	1 cup	100	0.0	0.6
Nutri-Grain, Corn	1 cup	160	1.0	2.6
Ripple Crisp Honey Corn - General Mills	1 cup	147	0.7	1.0
Sugar Corn Pops - Kellogg's	1 cup	110	0.0	1.0
Toasties, Corn Flakes	1 serv.	111	0.0	1.0
Total Corn Flakes - General Mills	1 cup	83	0.4	0.4

Rice Cereals

ITEM NAME	PORTION	CAL	FAT	FIBER
Crisp Rice, Low Sodium	1 cup	105	0.1	0.4
Crispy Rice	1 cup	112	0.1	1.0

ITEM NAME	PORTION	CAL	FAT	FIBER
Frosted Rice	1 cup	108	0.1	0.1
Lites, Puffed Rice - Health Valley	1 cup	100	0.0	0.7
Nutty Rice - Pacific Grain	1 cup	420	3.0	4.0
Rice, Puffed, Added Sugar	1 cup	115	0.0	0.2
Rice Chex - Ralston	1 cup	100	0.1	0.2
Rice Flakes	1 cup	124	0.1	0.4
Rice Krispies - Kellogg's	1 cup	88	0.0	0.8

Oat Cereals

ITEM NAME	PORTION	CAL	FAT	FIBER
✔ 100% Natural Oats & Honey - Quaker	1 cup	440	16.0	6.0
✔ Balance/Raisins & Rolled Oats	1 cup	224	1.8	7.3
Cheerios - General Mills	1 cup	110	2.0	3.0
Apple Cinnamon - General Mills	1 cup	160	3.3	1.3
Honey Nut - General Mills	1 cup	120	1.5	2.0
✔ Cinnamon Oat Squares - Quaker	1 cup	230	2.5	5.0
Fortified Oat Flakes	1 cup	177	0.7	1.2
Honey Bunches of Oats - Post	1 cup	160	2.0	1.3
Life, Oat/Cinnamon - Quaker	1 cup	190	2.0	3.0
Oat Squares - Quaker	1 cup	220	3.0	4.0
Oatmeal Crisp with Almonds - General Mills	1 cup	230	6.0	3.0
Oatmeal Crisp with Apples - General Mills	1 cup	210	2.5	3.0
Oatmeal Crisp with Raisins - General Mills	1 cup	210	3.0	2.0
Popeye Oat'mmms	1 cup	120	2.0	2.0
Toasted Oat - Nature Valley	1 cup	333	13.3	4.0

Wheat Cereals

ITEM NAME	PORTION	CAL	FAT	FIBER
Crispy Wheats'n Raisins	1 cup	160	0.7	2.9
Frosted Flakes - Kellogg's	1 cup	160	0.0	0.0
✔ Frosted Mini Wheats, Reg & Bite Size - Kellogg's	1 cup	190	1.0	6.0
✔ Frosted Wheat Bites - Nabisco	1 cup	190	1.0	5.0
✔ Fruit Wheats - Blueberry or Strawberry - Nabisco	1 cup	226	0.8	5.3
✔ Fruit Wheats - Raspberry - Nabisco	1 cup	226	0.8	5.3
✔ Grape Nuts - Post	½ cup	200	1.0	5.0
Grape Nuts Flakes - Post	1 cup	133	1.3	4.0
Lites, Puffed Wheat - Health Valley	1 cup	100	0.0	2.8
Mini Wheats/Brown Sugar Frosting	1 cup	176	0.5	4.6
✔ Nutri Grain, Golden Wheat - Kellogg's	1 cup	133	0.7	5.3
✔ Raisin Wheats	1 cup	217	0.4	6.0
✔ Shredded Wheat Biscuit Barbara's	2 items	140	1.0	5.0

13

ITEM NAME	PORTION	CAL	FAT	FIBER
✔ Nabisco Shredded Wheat, Spoon Size	2 pieces	160	0.5	5.0
✔ Nabisco	1 cup	170	0.5	5.0
✔ Barbara's	1 cup	160	2.0	6.0
✔ Shredded Wheat 'n Bran, Spoon Size-Nabisco	1 cup	194	0.6	7.4
Special K - Kellogg's	1 cup	110	0.0	1.0
Team - Nabisco	1 cup	176	0.0	0.8
Wheat, Puffed - Quaker	1 box	35	0.0	1.0
Wheat Chex	1 cup	169	1.1	3.4
Wheat Flakes, Added Sugar	1 cup	105	0.0	2.7
Wheat Germ - Kretschmer Honey Crunch	2 tbsp.	60	1.2	1.2
Wheaties - General Mills	1 cup	110	1.0	3.3
Wheaties Honey Gold - General Mills	1 cup	147	0.7	1.3
Whole Wheat Natural	1 cup	150	1.0	2.7

Multi-Grain Combinations & Others

ITEM NAME	PORTION	CAL	FAT	FIBER
100% Natural, Plain	1 cup	489	22.4	3.8
✔ 100% Natural Low Fat Crispy Whole Grain with Raisins - Quaker	1 cup	380	6.0	6.0
✔ Alpen - Muesli	1 cup	453	9.5	11.1
Alpha Bits - Post	1 cup	130	1.0	1.0
✔ Amaranth Flakes, Organic - Health Valley	1 cup	133	0.0	5.3
Apple Jacks - Kellogg's	1 cup	110	0.0	1.0
Apple Raisin Crisp - Kellogg's	1 cup	180	0.0	4.0
✔ Balance	1 cup	212	1.3	7.7
Banana Nut Crunch - Post	1 cup	250	6.0	4.0
Barbie, Sweetened - Ralston	1 cup	110	1.0	0.0
Basic Four - General Mills	1 cup	210	3.0	3.0
Blueberry Morning - Post	1 cup	184	2.8	1.6
Body Buddies, Natural Fruit - General Mills	1 cup	110	1.0	1.0
Booberry - General Mills	1 cup	120	0.5	0.5
C.W. Post, Plain	1 cup	432	15.2	2.2
C.W. Post, with Raisins	1 cup	446	14.7	2.0
✔ C.W. Post Hearty Granola	1 cup	372	12.0	5.3
Cap'n Crunch - Quaker	1 cup	133	2.0	1.3
Crunchberries - Quaker	1 cup	133	2.0	1.3
Peanut Butter - Quaker	1 cup	147	3.3	1.3
Cheerios, Multi-Grain - General Mills	1 cup	110	1.0	3.0
Chex				
✔ 100% Whole Wheat - Ralston	1 cup	253	1.0	7.0

ITEM NAME	PORTION	CAL	FAT	FIBER
Double Chex - Ralston	1 cup	96	0.0	0.0
Graham - Ralston	1 cup	210	2.0	1.0
Cinnamon Toast Crunch -				
General Mills	1 cup	160	3.9	1.3
Clusters - General Mills	1 cup	220	4.5	4.0
Coco Crunchies	1 cup	154	0.7	0.6
Cocoa Krispies - Kellogg's	1 cup	160	0.7	0.0
Cocoa Pebbles - Post	1 cup	160	1.3	1.0
Cocoa Puffs - General Mills	1 cup	120	1.0	0.2
Cookie Crisp - Ralston	1 cup	120	1.5	0.4
Count Chocula - General Mills	1 cup	117	0.4	0.6
Crispix - Kellogg's	1 cup	110	0.0	1.0
Crispy Critters - Post	1 serv.	110	0.0	1.0
✔ Fiber One - General Mills	½ cup	60	1.0	13.0
Fiber 7 Flakes - Health Valley	1 cup	133	0.0	5.3
✔ Fibre Crunch	1 cup	246	9.3	11.6
✔ Fibre One	½ cup	101	1.1	15.8
✔ Fibre Up	½ cup	65	0.4	13.8
Frankenberry - General Mills	1 cup	120	0.5	0.5
Froot Loops				
General Mills	1 cup	111	0.5	0.3
Kellogg's	1 cup	120	1.0	1.0
Frosted Flakes - Ralston	1 cup	149	0.5	0.8
Fruit & Fibre - Post				
✔ Cinnamon Apple Crisp	1 cup	143	1.7	6.0
✔ Dates, Raisins, Walnuts	1 cup	210	3.0	6.0
✔ Peach, Raisins, Almonds	1 cup	210	3.0	6.0
Pineapple, Banana	1 cup	161	2.7	6.5
Fruity Marshmallow Krispies	1 cup	106	0.1	0.2
Golden Grahams - General Mills	1 cup	160	1.3	1.3
Granola				
✔ Fat Free, Date & Almond/				
Tropical Fruit/Raisin				
Cinnamon - Health Valley	1 cup	270	0.0	9.0
Fruits & Nuts - Nature Valley	1 cup	375	16.5	4.5
✔ Homemade	½ cup	297	16.6	6.4
✔ Low Fat, Cinnamon/Raisins -				
General Mills	1 cup	420	5.0	6.0
Nature Valley	1 cup	320	10.7	4.0
✔ Sun Country Almond	1 cup	540	18.0	6.0
✔ Sun Country Raisin & Date	1 cup	520	16.0	8.0
Granola O's, Almond or				
Apple/Cinnamon - Health				
Valley	1 cup	160	0.0	4.0
✔ Great Grains Raisins, Dates				
& Pecans - Post	1 cup	315	7.5	6.0

ITEM NAME	PORTION	CAL	FAT	FIBER
Harvest Crunch	½ cup	242	11.1	2.8
Apples & Cinnamon	½ cup	212	8.9	3.3
Raisins & Dates	½ cup	255	10.7	3.3
Tropical Fruit	½ cup	217	8.8	2.8
Healthy Choice				
Multi-Grain Flakes	1 cup	100	0.0	3.0
Multi-Grain Squares	1 cup	152	0.8	4.8
✔ Heartland Natural, Plain	1 cup	499	17.7	5.4
Honey Almond Delight - Ralston	1 cup	210	3.0	4.0
✔ Honey Clusters & Flakes -				
Health Valley	1 cup	173	0.0	5.3
Honeycomb - Post	1 cup	83	0.0	0.2
Just Right Fruit & Nut - Kellogg's	1 cup	200	2.0	3.0
Kaboom - General Mills	1 cup	96	1.2	0.8
King Vitaman - Quaker	1 cup	80	0.7	0.7
Kix - General Mills	1 cup	90	0.8	1.0
Kix - Berry Berry, General Mills	1 cup	160	2.0	1.0
Life - Quaker	1 cup	160	2.0	2.7
Lucky Charms - General Mills	1 cup	120	1.0	1.0
Muesli				
✔ Banana Walnut - Ralston	1 cup	267	4.0	5.0
Blueberry Pecan - Ralston	1 cup	200	3.0	4.0
✔ Cranberry - Ralston	1 cup	267	4.0	5.0
✔ Mueslix Crispy Blend - Kellogg's	1 cup	300	4.5	6.0
✔ Mueslix Golden Crunch - Kellogg's	1 cup	280	6.7	8.0
Nutri-Grain				
Almond Raisin	1 cup	160	2.4	3.2
Barley	1 cup	153	0.3	2.4
Rye	1 cup	144	0.3	2.6
Nutri Grain Cereal Bar, Blueberry -				
Kellogg's	1 bar	140	4.0	1.0
✔ Nutri Grain Nuggets	1 cup	360	2.0	14.0
Oh's, Honey Graham - Quaker	1 cup	147	2.7	1.3
Oh's, Honey Nut - Quaker	1 cup	197	6.3	1.4
Pac Man	1 cup	120	0.5	0.6
Pep	1 cup	129	0.4	3.8
Pro Stars	1 cup	95	0.8	0.9
Product 19 - Kellogg's	1 cup	110	0.0	1.0
✔ Shreddies & Raisins	1 cup	208	0.5	5.6
S'mores Grahams - General Mills	1 cup	160	2.0	1.0
✔ Squares: Apple Cinnamon,				
Blueberry, & Raisin - Kellogg's	1 cup	240	1.3	6.7
✔ Squares: Strawberry - Kellogg's	1 cup	180	1.0	5.0
✔ Strawberry Wheats	1 cup	234	0.8	5.9
Sugar Crisp	1 cup	124	0.4	1.0
Sugar Smacks - Kellogg's	1 cup	147	0.7	1.3

ITEM NAME	PORTION	CAL	FAT	FIBER
Sun Crunchers - General Mills	1 cup	210	3.0	3.0
Sun Flakes, Corn & Rice - Ralston	1 cup	147	1.0	1.0
Super Sugar Crisp - Post	1 cup	123	0.3	0.5
Tasteeos	1 cup	94	0.7	0.8
Toasties - Post	1 cup	100	0.0	1.0
Total - General Mills	1 cup	147	1.3	4.0
Triples - General Mills	1 cup	120	1.0	0.8
Trix - General Mills	1 cup	120	1.5	0.3
Weetabix	1 cup	108	0.6	3.7

Hot Cereals

ITEM NAME	PORTION	CAL	FAT	FIBER
Apple Raisin Spice - Pritikin	1 packet	170	2.5	4.0
✔ Bear Mush, Creamy Wheat - Arrowhead Mills	1 cup	640	4.0	8.0
Corn Grits, White or Yellow	1 cup	560	2.0	4.0
Cream of Rice, Cooked	1 cup	127	0.2	0.4
Cream of Wheat	1 packet	130	0.4	2.0
Cream of Wheat, Instant	1 cup	153	0.6	2.2
Cream of Wheat, Regular, Hot	1 cup	103	0.5	1.9
Cream of Wheat/Iron, Quick, Cooked	1 cup	133	0.4	1.7
Farina, Enriched - Country Choice	1 cup	100	0.0	0.8
✔ Oat Bran	1 cup	204	5.0	10.9
Raisin/Cinnamon - Quaker	1 serv.	120	2.0	3.0
Regular Flavor - Quaker	1 serv.	100	2.0	4.0
Malt O Meal, Cooked	1 cup	122	0.3	0.6
✔ Maltex, Hot Wheat Cereal	1 cup	510	1.0	15.0
✔ Maypo, Instant Hot Cereal - Maple	1 cup	380	4.0	6.0
✔ Mother's Instant Oatmeal	1 cup	300	6.0	8.0
✔ Mother's Oat Bran	1 cup	300	6.0	12.0
✔ Mother's Multigrain	1 cup	260	3.0	10.0
✔ Mother's Whole Wheat	1 cup	260	2.0	8.0
Multigrain - Pritikin	1 packet	160	1.5	4.0
✔ Oat Bran, Cooked - Quaker	1 cup	300	6.0	12.0
Oatmeal, Cooked	1 cup	145	2.4	4.5
Oatmeal, Instant				
Apples & Cinnamon - Quaker	1 packet	130	1.5	3.0
Cinnamon-Spice - Quaker	1 packet	170	2.0	3.0
Maple/Brown Sugar - Quaker	1 packet	160	2.0	3.0
Peaches & Cream - Quaker	1 packet	130	2.0	2.0
✔ Oats, Old Fashioned & Quick, Uncooked - Quaker	1 cup	300	6.0	8.0
✔ Rice and Shine, Organic - Arrowhead Mills	1 cup	600	4.0	8.0
Roman Meal, Cooked	1 cup	147	1.0	2.3
✔ Seven Grain, Organic - Arrowhead Mills	1 cup	420	4.5	15.0

ITEM NAME	PORTION	CAL	FAT	FIBER
Wheat, Ralston	1 cup	134	0.8	4.2
Wheat Hearts - General Mills	1 cup	130	9.0	2.0

PANCAKES

(There are typically 3 four-inch pancakes in a serving)

Blueberry				
Microwave - Pillsbury	1 serv.	230	4.0	1.0
Mix - Bisquick	1 serv.	270	3.0	0.9
Mix - Hungry Jack	1 serv.	170	1.0	0.9
Buckwheat, Mix	1 serv.	165	6.0	1.8
Buttermilk				
Mix - Betty Crocker	3 pncks.	200	3.0	1.0
Mix - Hungry Jack	1 serv.	180	1.0	0.5
Microwave - Pillsbury	1 serv.	260	4.0	1.0
Mix - Bisquick	1 serv.	250	3.0	0.7
✓ Oat Bran, Lite - Krusteaz	3 pncks.	140	1.0	7.0
Oat Bran, Microwave - Pillsbury	1 serv.	230	4.0	3.0
Original, Complete, Mix -				
Betty Crocker	3 pncks.	210	3.0	1.0
Original, Microwave - Pillsbury	1 serv.	240	2.0	2.0
Original, Mix - Bisquick	1 serv.	250	3.0	3.0
Soybean, 25% Soy Flour, Mix	1 serv.	68	1.9	0.5
Wheat, Microwave - Pillsbury	1 serv.	240	4.0	4.2
Whole Wheat, Microwave -				
Pillsbury	1 serv.	230	4.0	3.0

WAFFLES & FRENCH TOAST

Waffles				
Buttermilk, Frozen - Aunt				
Jemima	1 item	95	3.0	0.5
Home Recipe	1 item	245	12.6	1.1
Nutri Grain Multi Bran - Eggo/				
Kellogg's	1 item	90	3.0	3.0
✓ Oat Bran - Belgian Chef	1 item	80	3.0	6.0
Oat Bran, No Cholesterol -				
Eggo/Kellogg's	1 item	100	3.5	1.5
Oatmeal, Frozen - Aunt Jemima	1 item	100	4.0	2.0
Raisin Bran, Nutri Grain -				
Eggo/Kellogg's	1 item	105	3.0	2.5
French Toast				
Frozen - Campbells	1 slice	94	5.0	1.6
Home Recipe	1 slice	153	6.7	2.0
Sourdough, Frozen - Krusteaz	1 slice	140	2.0	0.0

DAIRY PRODUCTS

Dairy products do not contain any fiber. There may be some fiber, though, in yogurts to which fruits and grains have been added. In addition, there are some cocoa mixes that contain small amounts of fiber.

ITEM NAME	PORTION	CAL	FAT	FIBER
Cheeses & Cheese spreads (Cheese Only), All Varieties	—	—	—	0.0
Cream, Sour, Half & Half, & Whipping	—	—	—	0.0
Junket (Rennet Custard), Made with Nonfat Dry Milk	1 cup	176	<1.0	0.2
Junket (Rennet Custard), Made with Whole Milk	1 cup	280	9.0	0.3
Malted, Dry Powder	1 tbsp.	86	2.0	0.1
Milk,				
Whole, 2%, or skim, Nonflavored (fat and calories will change with the different nonflavored milks, but the fiber remains zero)	1 cup	—	—	0.0
Chocolate, 1% Fat	1 cup	158	3.0	0.2
Chocolate, Hot, Homemade	1 cup	250	13.0	0.3
Chocolate - Nestle Quick	1 cup	230	9.0	0.0
Malted, Natural Flavor	1 cup	236	10.0	0.1
Milk Shake				
Chocolate, Thick	1 cup	413	9.0	0.9
Vanilla, Thick	1 cup	386	11.0	0.2
Yogurt				
Breakfast, Tropical Fruit (6 oz. cup)	1 item	210	3.0	2.0
Light 'n Crunchy, Raspberry Granola - Dannon	1 item	150	0.0	2.0
Plain, Low Fat - Dannon	1 cup	240	3.0	1.0
Plain, Non-Fat - Yoplait	1 cup	210	0.0	0.0
Strawberry Banana - Weight Watchers	1 cup	90	0.0	2.0
Strawberry Crunch/Granola (7 oz. cup) - Yoplait	1 item	130	1.0	4.0

ENTREES & MEAL COMBINATIONS

At the top of this category's fiber list you'll find those meat, poultry, salad, and rice-based foods that contain fiber-rich legumes, such as beans, lentils, and peas. There's also a lot of fiber to be found in vegetable-based entrees, and vegetarian entrees that are designed to resemble meat/poultry dishes. You'll find some variation in the fiber content of pastas and pizzas, all dependent on the types of sauces and ingredients being used. Note that even the most fibrous and dense meats contain no fiber that can be used by your body.

ITEM NAME	PORTION	CAL	FAT	FIBER
Meat only, including beef and pork, all cuts and preparations including baking, frying, roasting, and broiling	—	—	—	0.0

FOODS CONTAINING MEAT

ITEM NAME	PORTION	CAL	FAT	FIBER
ABCs & 123s, Mini Meatballs - Chef Boyardee	1 cup	280	9.0	4.0
✔ Beans & Wieners, Beanee Weenee - Van Camp's	1 cup	405	18.0	10.5
Beef Chow Mein/Chop Suey w/Noodles	1 cup	465	25.0	3.5
Beef Potpie, Home Recipe - 1/3 of 9" Pie	1 slice	515	30.0	3.9
Beef Ravioli, Tomato & Meat Sauce - Chef Boyardee	1 cup	230	5.0	4.0
Beef Stew - Dinty Moore	1 cup	230	14.0	2.0
Beef Stew with Vegetables	1 cup	220	11.0	3.2
✔ Beefaroni - Chef Boyardee	1 cup	280	7.0	5.0
Beefogetti, Pasta/Mini Meatballs in Sauce - Chef Boyardee	1 cup	250	10.0	3.0
Cheese Ravioli/Tomato Sauce/Beef - Chef Boyardee	1 cup	220	3.0	4.0
Chompsalot Cheese Ravioli/Meat Sauce - Chef Boyardee	1 cup	210	4.0	4.0
Chili				
✔ Beef & Beans - Hormel	1 cup	340	17.0	9.0
✔ Classic with Beans - Stagg	1 cup	330	15.0	14.0
✔ Con Carne w/Beans - Nalley	1 cup	290	9.0	13.0
No Beans - Hormel	1 cup	410	30.0	3.0
Steak House - Stagg	1 cup	360	22.0	13.0
✔ Chili Mac, Macaroni w/Beef in Chili - Chef Boyardee	1 cup	260	11.0	8.0
Chimichanga, Beef	1 item	425	20.0	4.3
Corn Dog, Plain	1 item	460	19.0	2.8
Corned Beef Hash				
✔ Libby's	1 cup	490	36.0	9.0
Enchirito, Cheese/Beef/Bean	1 item	344	16.0	3.4

ITEM NAME	PORTION	CAL	FAT	FIBER
Fajita, Beef	1 serv.	244	10.0	2.2
Fettuccine, Hearty Meat Sauce -				
Chef Boyardee	1 cup	230	6.0	4.0
Hot Dog, Plain with Bun	1 item	242	15.0	0.9
✔ Lasagna, Pasta and Beef Sauce -				
Chef Boyardee	1 cup	270	11.0	5.0
Meatloaf, with Celery and Onions	1 serv.	213	14.0	0.1
Mini Beef Ravioli in Tomato/				
Meat Sauce - Chef Boyardee	1 cup	230	5.0	4.0
Mini Cannelloni (Beef) in				
Meat Sauce - Chef Boyardee	1 cup	260	9.0	4.0
MiniBites, Cheese Ravioli/				
Meatballs/Sauce - Chef Boyardee	1 cup	270	11.0	3.0
Peas				
✔ Blackeye & Corn, Seasoned/				
Pork - Luck's	1 cup	260	6.0	6.0
✔ Crowder, Seasoned/Pork -				
Luck's	1 cup	240	6.0	8.0
✔ Field w/Snap Beans,				
Seasoned/Pork - Luck's	1 cup	260	6.0	8.0
Peppers, Sweet, Red & Green,				
Beef & Crumbs	1 cup	238	8.0	2.2
Pork & Beans				
✔ Baked Canned	1 cup	268	4.0	14.0
✔ with Frankfurters, Canned	1 cup	365	17.0	12.8
✔ Great Northern, Seasoned -				
Luck's	1 cup	280	6.0	12.0
✔ Kidney, Red - Luck's	1 cup	280	5.0	14.0
✔ Lima, Giant, Seasoned - Luck's	1 cup	300	6.0	10.0
✔ Mixed Pinto & Northern - Luck's	1 cup	260	5.0	12.0
✔ Navy, Seasoned - Luck's	1 cup	280	8.0	10.0
✔ Pinto, Seasoned - Luck's	1 cup	280	8.0	12.0
✔ in Sweet Sauce, Canned	1 cup	281	4.0	14.0
✔ in Tomato Sauce, Canned -				
Van Camp's	1 cup	220	3.0	12.0
Pork Chow Mein/Chop Suey				
w/Noodles	1 oz.	56	3.0	0.4
Ravioli, Beef & Garlic, Fresh -				
Contadina	1 cup	280	11.0	2.4
Rigatoni, Macaroni in Tomato/				
Meat Sauce - Chef Boyardee	1 cup	250	7.0	4.0
✔ Roller Coasters, Pasta/Meatballs				
in Sauce - Chef Boyardee	1 cup	260	11.0	5.0
Salmon Rice Loaf	1 cup	256	10.0	0.7
Sharks Pasta with Mini Meatballs -				
Chef Boyardee	1 cup	260	9.0	4.0

ITEM NAME	PORTION	CAL	FAT	FIBER
Sir Chompsalot Lasagna w/Meatballs - Chef Boyardee	1 cup	210	3.0	4.0
Sir Chompsalot Pasta Rings w/Meatballs - Chef Boyardee	1 cup	280	10.0	4.0
Spaghetti/Tomato/Meat - Home Recipe	1 cup	330	12.0	2.7
Spaghetti/Tomato/Meat, Canned	1 cup	260	10.0	2.8
Spaghetti & Meatballs in Tomato Sauce - Chef Boyardee	1 cup	250	10.0	3.0
✔ Spaghettio's/Meatballs - Franco-American	1 cup	260	11.0	5.0
Spaghettio's/Sliced Franks - Franco-American	1 cup	250	11.0	4.0
Sportyo's Pasta/Meatballs/Sauce - Franco-American	1 oz.	29	1.0	0.4
Stew, Brunswick, Microwave - Luck's	1 serv.	150	1.0	3.0
Tamales, Beef				
Gebhardt	1 item	112	8.0	2.2
Hormel	1 item	93	7.0	1.0
Teenage Ninja Turtles/Meatballs in Sauce - Chef Boyardee	1 cup	260	3.0	4.0
Tic Tac Toes with Mini Meatballs - Chef Boyardee	1 cup	260	10.0	4.0
Tortellini, Chicken & Vegetable - Contadina	1 cup	347	9.0	2.7
✔ Tortellini in Meat Sauce - Chef Boyardee	1 cup	260	3.0	8.0
Tortelloni, Sweet Italian Sausage - Contadina	1 cup	330	10.0	3.0
Tortelloni, Chicken & Prosciutto - Contadina	1 cup	360	13.0	3.0
✔ Turnip Greens & Diced Turnips, Seasoned/Pork - Luck's	1 cup	180	10.0	8.0
Welsh Rarebit	1 cup	399	30.0	0.1

FOODS CONTAINING POULTRY, EGGS, OR FISH

ITEM NAME	PORTION	CAL	FAT	FIBER
Chicken, Turkey, Duck, Fish (flesh only) all types, cuts and preparations including baking, frying, roasting and broiling	1 serv.	—	—	0.0
Eggs & egg substitutes	1 serv.	—	—	0.0
Chicken a la King, Cooked - Home Recipe	1 cup	470	34.0	1.2
Chicken & Cashew Take Out Cuisine - House of Tsang	1 serv.	440	17.0	2.0

ITEM NAME	PORTION	CAL	FAT	FIBER
Chicken & Dumplings - Luck's	1 serv.	260	12.0	4.0
Microwave - Luck's	1 serv.	170	2.0	2.0
Chicken & Potatoes, Microwave - Luck's	1 serv.	190	4.0	3.0
Chicken & Rice, Microwave - Luck's	1 serv.	150	2.0	2.0
Chicken Chow Mein				
Canned - Chun King	1 cup	100	3.0	4.0
Home Recipe	1 cup	255	10.0	0.5
Take Out Cuisine - House of Tsang	1 serv.	350	13.0	1.0
Chicken Potpie, Baked - Home Recipe	1 slice	545	31.0	4.2
Fajita - Chicken	1 serv.	170	3.0	2.2
Fish				
Haddock, Breaded, Fried	1 piece	140	5.0	0.3
Shrimp, French Fried	1 serv.	206	10.0	0.5
Salmon Rice Loaf	1 serv.	122	5.0	0.7
Fish Cakes, Fried	1 cup	361	17.0	2.5
Plate Dinner, Chicken, Fried, Potatoes	1 cup	431	21.0	2.6
Sweet & Sour Chicken, Take Out Cuisine - House of Tsang	1 serv.	410	8.0	2.0
Tamales, Chicken & Cheese - Trader Joe's	1 item	270	13.0	3.0
Turkey Chili - Hormel	1 cup	190	3.0	3.0
Turkey Pot Pie				
Baked, Home, Prepared	1 cup	569	32.0	2.8
Frozen	1 cup	473	25.0	2.7

PASTA-BASED COMBINATIONS

ITEM NAME	PORTION	CAL	FAT	FIBER
ABC's & 123's in Sauce - Chef Boyardee	1 serv.	160	1.0	3.0
Cheese Ravioli in Sauce - Chef Boyardee	1 cup	210	0.0	4.0
Dinosaurs, Tomato/Cheese Flavored Sauce - Chef Boyardee	1 cup	210	0.0	3.0
Lasagna, 7.5 oz. - Chef Boyardee	1 serv.	240	8.0	3.2
Macaroni & Cheese				
Chef Boyardee	1 cup	210	3.0	2.0
Home Recipe	1 cup	430	22.0	1.2
Kraft	1 cup	260	3.0	1.0
Macaroni Shells - Chef Boyardee	1 serv.	150	1.0	1.7
Mini Bites - Chef Boyardee	1 serv.	260	12.0	1.0

ITEM NAME	PORTION	CAL	FAT	FIBER
✔ Mini Cannelloni - Chef Boyardee	1 serv.	230	7.0	5.0
Ninja Turtles, Tomato/Cheese Flavored Sauce - Chef Boyardee	1 cup	170	0.0	3.0
Noodles				
Alfredo & Sauce - Farmhouse	1 cup	260	4.0	2.0
Creamy Chicken/Sauce - Farmhouse	1 cup	240	2.0	2.0
Herb/Butter & Sauce - Farmhouse	1 cup	240	2.0	1.0
Parmesano & Sauce - Farmhouse	1 cup	260	3.0	2.0
Stroganoff & Sauce - Farmhouse	1 cup	240	3.0	2.0
Pasta in Pizza Sauce, PizzaO's - Franco-American	1 cup	210	3.0	2.0
Roller Coaster - Chef Boyardee	1 serv.	230	10.0	3.0
Sharks, Tomato and Cheese Flavored Sauce - Chef Boyardee	1 cup	160	0.0	3.0
✔ Sir Chompsalot Ravioli, Tomato/ Cheese Sauce - Chef Boyardee	1 cup	210	0.0	5.0
Smurf - Chef Boyardee	1 serv.	150	1.0	3.0
✔ Smurf Ravioli, Pasta/Sauce - Chef Boyardee	1 serv.	230	5.0	6.3
✔ Spaghetti, Tomato Sauce, Cheese, Canned	1 cup	190	2.0	7.8
Spaghetti, Tomato/Cheese				
Canned	1 cup	190	2.0	2.5
Home Recipe	1 cup	260	9.0	2.5
Teddyo's in Cheese Sauce - Franco-American	1 cup	190	2.0	2.0
Tic Tac Toes - Chef Boyardee	1 serv.	160	1.0	3.0
Tic Tac Toes, Pasta-Tomato/ Cheese Flavored Sauce - Chef Boyardee	1 cup	190	0.0	3.0
✔ Tortellini, Cheese in Tomato Sauce - Chef Boyardee	1 cup	230	1.0	5.0
Tortellini, Cheese, Fresh - Contadina	1 cup	347	8.0	3.0

NON-MEAT FOODS

ITEM NAME	PORTION	CAL	FAT	FIBER
✔ Amaranth/Fast Menu, Fat Free - Health Valley	1 cup	160	0.0	9.0
Beans				
Chili - S&W	1 cup	220	2.0	12.0

ITEM NAME	PORTION	CAL	FAT	FIBER
✔ Mexican Pinto/Rice, Cooked - Farmhouse	1 cup	190	1.0	6.0
Red, & Rice, Cooked - Farmhouse	1 cup	180	1.0	4.0
✔ Spanish Black/Rice, Cooked - Farmhouse	1 cup	200	1.0	6.0
Big Franks, Meatless - Loma Linda	1 link	110	7.0	2.0
✔ Burrito, Beans and Cheese	1 item	189	6.0	8.3
Cheese Souffle - Home Recipe	1 cup	207	16.0	0.1
Chicken Supreme, Meatless - Loma Linda	⅓ cup	90	1.0	4.0
Chili				
✔ Black Bean	1 cup	160	0.0	14.0
✔ Canned - Worthington	1 cup	290	15.0	9.0
✔ Vegetarian, Canned - Natural Touch	1 cup	270	12.0	11.0
✔ Vegetarian, Mild w/Beans - Health Valley	1 cup	160	0.0	14.0
✔ Vegetarian, Spicy w/Black Beans - Health Valley	1 cup	160	0.0	14.0
✔ Vegetarian Quick Meal - Spice Islands	1 pkg.	180	2.0	7.0
with Beans - Chili Bowl	1 oz.	30	2.0	0.6
✔ with Beans, Canned	1 cup	286	14.0	6.9
Choplets, Canned - Worthington	2 slices	90	2.0	2.0
Chow Mein, Canned - La Choy	1 cup	69	<1.0	0.2
Chow Mein Vegetables, Canned - Chun King	1 cup	20	0.0	2.0
✔ Country Stew, Canned - Worthington	1 cup	210	9.0	5.0
Cutlets, Canned - Worthington	1 slice	70	1.0	2.0
Diced Chik, Canned - Worthington	¼ cup	60	4.0	1.0
Dinner Cuts, Meatless, Canned - Loma Linda	1 slice	80	2.0	3.0
Enchilada, Cheese	1 item	320	19.0	3.2
Falafel, Mix - Casbah	5 balls	130	3.0	2.0
FriChik, Canned - Worthington	2 pieces	120	8.0	1.0
Fried Chik'n n/Gravy, Canned - Loma Linda	2 pieces	390	31	3.0
Granburger, Dry - Worthington	3 tbsp.	60	1.0	2.0
Hummus, Mix - Casbah	½ cup	240	10.0	2.0
Little Links, Canned - Loma Linda	2 links	90	6.0	2.0
✔ Loaf Mix, Dry - Natural Touch	4 tbsp.	100	1.0	7.0
Multigrain Cutlet, Canned - Worthington	2 slices	100	2.0	4.0
Nachos, Cheese	1 serv.	345	19.0	2.2

ITEM NAME	PORTION	CAL	FAT	FIBER
Numete, ³/₈" Slices, Canned - Worthington	1 slice	130	10.0	3.0
Nuteena, Canned, ³/₈" Slices - La Loma	1 slice	160	13.0	2.0
Ocean Platter, Dry - La Loma	¹/₃ cup	90	1.0	4.0
Pasta Vegetarian Cuisine				
Linguini Primavera, Fat Free - Health Valley	1 cup	110	0.0	3.0
Pasta Fagioli - Health Valley	1 cup	120	0.0	4.0
Spicy Rotini - Health Valley	1 cup	100	0.0	4.0
✔ Patty Mix, Dry - La Loma	¹/₃ cup	90	1.0	5.0
Potato, Au Gratin - Home Recipe	1 cup	323	19.0	4.4
Prime Steaks, Canned - Worthington	1 piece	140	9.0	4.0
Protose, ³/₈" Slices, Canned - Worthington	1 slice	130	7.0	3.0
Redi-Burger, ⁵/₈" Slices, Canned - Loma Linda	1 slice	170	10.0	4.0
✔ Rotini/Vegetables - Pasta Perfect	1 cup	220	2.0	5.2
Sandwich Spread, Canned - La Loma	¹/₄ cup	80	5.0	3.0
Saucettes, Canned - Worthington	1 link	90	6.0	1.0
✔ Savory Dinner Loaf Mix, Dry - La Loma	¹/₃ cup	90	2.0	5.0
Savory Slices, Canned - Worthington	3 slices	150	9.0	3.0
Sliced Chik, Canned - Worthington	3 slices	90	6.0	1.0
Soyagen All Purpose, Dry - Loma Linda	¹/₄ cup	130	6.0	3.0
Spinach Souffle	1 cup	219	18.0	0.8
Stroganoff Mix, Dry - Natural Touch	4 tbsp.	90	4.0	3.0
Super Links, Canned - Worthington	1 link	110	8.0	1.0
Swiss Steak, Canned - Loma Linda	1 piece	120	6.0	4.0
Taco	1 item	370	21.0	2.7
Taco Mix, Dry - Natural Touch	3 tbsp.	60	1.0	3.0
Tamale, Green Chile & Cheese - Trader Joe's	1 item	270	17.0	4.0
Tender Bits, Canned - Loma Linda	6 pieces	110	5.0	3.0
Tender Rounds, Canned - Loma Linda	8 pieces	120	5.0	3.0
Tofu Fast Menu				
✔ Baked Beans/Tofu Wieners - Health Valley	1 cup	170	1.0	16.0
✔ Black Beans & Vegetables - Health Valley	1 cup	230	1.0	19.0
✔ Lentils & Vegetables - Health Valley	1 cup	160	1.0	12.0

ITEM NAME	PORTION	CAL	FAT	FIBER
Turkey Slices, Canned - Worthington	3 slices	190	14.0	2.0
Vege Burger, Canned - Loma Linda	¼ cup	70	2.0	2.0
Vegetable Skallops, Canned - Worthington	½ cup	90	2.0	3.0
Vegetable Steaks, Canned - Worthington	2 pieces	80	2.0	3.0
Vita-Burger, Dry - Loma Linda	¼ cup	70	1.0	3.0

"HELPER" COMBINATIONS

(serving size reflects portion of prepared dish)

Chicken Helper

	PORTION	CAL	FAT	FIBER
Stirfried Chicken, Skillet	1 cup	14	1.0	1.0

Hamburger Helper

Alfredo	1 cup	150	4.0	0.8
Beef Noodle	1 cup	120	2.0	0.8
Beef Taco	1 cup	150	2.0	0.8
Beef Teriyaki	1 cup	170	1.0	0.8
Cheddar 'n Bacon	1 cup	170	5.0	0.8
Cheeseburger Macaroni	1 cup	170	4.0	1.0
Chili Macaroni	1 cup	140	1.0	0.8
Hamburger Stew	1 cup	100	1.0	3.0
Lasagna	1 cup	140	1.0	1.0
Mushroom & Wild Rice	1 cup	170	3.0	0.8
Nacho Cheese	1 cup	160	3.0	0.8
Pizza Pasta with Cheese Topping	1 cup	150	2.0	1.0
Potatoes Au Gratin	1 cup	120	3.0	2.0
Spaghetti	1 cup	150	1.0	0.8
Stroganoff, Dry	1 cup	170	3.0	0.8
Three Cheese	1 cup	190	6.0	0.9
Zesty Italian	1 cup	160	1.0	0.8

Tuna Helper

Au Gratin	1 cup	190	4.0	1.0
Creamy Broccoli	1 cup	190	5.0	1.0
Creamy Noodle	1 cup	190	6.0	1.0
Fettuccine Alfredo	1 cup	180	4.0	0.9
Garden Cheddar	1 cup	190	4.0	1.0
Tetrazzini	1 cup	180	3.0	1.0
Tuna Pot Pie	1 pie	340	20.0	1.0
Tuna Romanoff	1 cup	210	3.0	1.0
Tuna Salad	1 cup	165	1.0	1.5

ITEM NAME	PORTION	CAL	FAT	FIBER
Pizza Combinations				
Beef, Thin 'N Crispy - Pizza Hut	1/8 med	229	11.0	2.0
Cheese, Pan (Thick) - Pizza Hut	1/8 med	261	11.0	2.0
Cheese, Thin 'N Crispy - Pizza Hut	1/8 med	205	8.0	2.0
Ham, Hand Tossed - Pizza Hut	1/8 med	213	5.0	2.0
Italian Sausage, Thin 'N Crispy - Pizza Hut	1/8 med	236	12.0	2.0
Meat Lover's, Pan (Thick) - Pizza Hut	1/8 med	340	18.0	2.0
Pepperoni				
Hand Tossed - Pizza Hut	1/8 med	238	8.0	2.0
Pan (Thick) - Pizza Hut	1/8 med	265	12.0	2.0
✔ Personal Pan - Pizza Hut	1 item	637	28.0	5.0
Thin 'N Crispy - Pizza Hut	1/8 med	215	10.0	1.0
Pork Topping, Hand Tossed - Pizza Hut	1/8 med	268	10.0	2.0
Super Supreme, Pan (Thick) - Pizza Hut	1/8 med	323	17.0	3.0
Supreme, Pan (Thick) - Pizza Hut	1/8 med	311	15.0	3.0
✔ Supreme, Personal Pan - Pizza Hut	1 item	722	34.0	6.0
Veggie Lover's, Pan (Thick) - Pizza Hut	1/8 med	243	10.0	3.0
Veggie Lover's, Hand Tossed - Pizza Hut	1/8 med	216	6.0	3.0
Rice Combinations (Cooked)				
Beef - Farmhouse	1 cup	200	1.0	2.0
Broccoli au Gratin - Farmhouse	1 cup	210	2.0	2.0
Broccoli au Gratin, Dry - Rice-a-Roni	1/3 cup	270	6.0	2.0
Chicken Pilaf - Farmhouse	1 cup	190	2.0	3.0
Chicken - Farmhouse	1 cup	180	2.0	4.0
Chicken & Broccoli, Dry - Rice-a-Roni	1/3 cup	240	2.0	2.0
Fried Rice, Dry - Rice-a-Roni	1/3 cup	240	2.0	2.0
Herb & Butter - Farmhouse	1 cup	210	2.0	2.0
Mexican - Farmhouse	1 cup	180	1.0	3.0
Oriental Fried - Farmhouse	1 cup	200	2.0	2.0
✔ Oriental & Vegetables Quick Meal - Spice Island	1 pkg.	180	3.0	13.0
Pilaf - Farmhouse	1 cup	200	1.0	2.0
Saffron Yellow - Farmhouse	1 cup	190	1.0	4.0
Spanish Rice, - Rice-a-Roni	1/3 cup	190	1.0	2.0
✔ Spicy Black Bean Quick Meal - Spice Island	1 pkg.	190	1.0	7.0

ITEM NAME	PORTION	CAL	FAT	FIBER
Traditional Long Grain & Wild - Farmhouse	1 cup	190	2.0	3.0
Whole Grain Quick Brown - Farmhouse	1 cup	160	2.0	3.0

SALADS				
Caesar - Suddenly Salad	1 cup	227	1.0	1.3
✓ Carrot Raisin - Home Recipe	1 cup	306	12.0	16.7
Chef, with Ham and Cheese	1 serv.	196	13.0	2.4
Chicken	1 cup	502	36.0	2.2
Classic Pasta - Suddenly Salad	1 cup	227	1.0	1.3
Coleslaw	1 tbsp.	6	0.0	0.3
Crab	1 serv.	145	9.0	0.3
Creamy Macaroni - Suddenly Salad	1 cup	195	1.0	1.5
Fruit, Canned, Water Pack	1 cup	74	<1.0	4.5
Gelatin, Mandarin Orange	1 serv.	23	0.0	0.6
Green Salad - Tossed	1 serv.	32	<1.0	2.1
Lobster with Tomato and Egg	1 cup	211	13.0	2.1
Macaroni	1 serv.	51	3.0	0.3
Pasta				
Creamy Dill - Kraft	1 cup	400	22.0	0.9
Garden Primavera - Kraft	1 cup	340	14.0	0.8
Herb & Garlic - Kraft	1 cup	420	24.0	1.0
Homestyle - Kraft	1 cup	480	32.0	1.9
Ranchers Choice - Kraft	1 cup	480	32.0	1.0
Ranch & Bacon - Suddenly Salad	1 cup	200	1.0	1.3
Taco	1 serv.	279	15.0	2.8
✓ Three Bean, Canned - Green Giant	1 cup	140	0.0	6.0
Tuna/Celery/Mayonnaise/Pickle/Egg	1 cup	350	22.0	1.0

FAST FOODS

Fiber in fast foods? It's there if you know where to look! The variety of foods available through fast food outlets has expanded in recent years. You can now order fiber-rich soups, salads, and vegetables, such as potatoes, carrot sticks, and corn-on-the-cob. In many cases, though, the only fiber to be found is in the breading of fat-laden, deep-fried foods.

ITEM NAME	PORTION	CAL	FAT	FIBER
ARBY'S				
Beef and Cheese Sandwich	1 item	508	26.5	1.1
Chicken Breast Sandwich	1 item	445	22.5	1.6

ITEM NAME	PORTION	CAL	FAT	FIBER
Club Sandwich	1 item	560	30.0	2.3
Ham and Cheese Sandwich	1 item	355	14.2	1.0
Roast Beef Sandwich	1 item	383	18.2	1.0
Soup				
Boston Clam Chowder	1 serv.	193	10.0	1.4
Cream of Broccoli	1 serv.	166	7.2	1.8
French Onion	1 serv.	67	3.0	0.9
Lumberjack Mixed Vegetable	1 serv.	89	3.6	1.3
Old Fashioned Chicken Noodle	1 serv.	99	1.8	0.7
Pilgrim Clam Chowder	1 serv.	193	11.0	1.9
Roast Beef and Vegetable	1 serv.	96	3.0	0.5
Split Pea and Ham	1 serv.	200	10.0	3.9
Tomato Florentine	1 serv.	84	2.0	0.5
Wisconsin Cheese	1 serv.	281	18.0	1.8
Super Roast Beef Sandwich	1 item	552	28.3	1.6

BURGER KING

ITEM NAME	PORTION	CAL	FAT	FIBER
Bacon Double Cheese, Deluxe	1 serv.	592	39.0	1.1
Barbecue Bacon Double Cheese	1 item	536	31.0	0.8
BK Broiler Sauce	1 serv.	90	10.0	0.0
Chicken, BK Broiler Chicken				
Sandwich	1 item	540	6.0	2.0
Chicken Tenders	1 piece	39	2.2	0.3
Croissant, Egg and Cheese	1 item	369	24.7	2.1
Double Cheeseburger	1 item	483	27.0	1.4
Fish, BK Big Fish Sandwich	1 item	720	8.0	2.0
Fish Tenders	1 serv.	267	16.0	1.1
Hamburger	1 item	330	15.0	1.0
with Cheese	1 item	380	19.0	1.0
Whopper	1 item	640	39.0	3.0
Whopper with Cheese	1 item	730	46.0	3.0
Whopper, Double	1 item	870	56.0	3.0
Whopper Jr.	1 item	420	24.0	2.0
Whopper Jr. with Cheese	1 item	460	28.0	2.0
Milk Shake, Chocolate, Medium	1 item	310	7.0	3.0
Milk Shake, Vanilla, Medium	1 item	310	7.0	1.0
✓ Onion Rings	1 serv.	310	14.0	5.0
Potatoes, Hash Brown	1 serv.	220	12.0	2.0
Salad, Garden	1 serv.	90	5.0	3.0
Salad, Side	1 serv.	50	3.0	2.0
Sweet & Sour Sauce	1 serv.	45	0.0	0.0
Tartar Dip Sauce	1 serv.	174	18.0	0.0

ITEM NAME	PORTION	CAL	FAT	FIBER
HARDEE				
Bacon & Egg Biscuit	1 serv.	410	24.0	0.6
Bacon Egg and Cheese Biscuit	1 serv.	460	28.0	0.7
Big Country Breakfast, with Bacon	1 serv.	660	40.0	0.0
Big Roast Beef Sandwich	1 serv.	300	11.0	0.9
Big Twin Hamburger	1 serv.	450	25.0	1.7
Grilled Chicken Sandwich	1 serv.	310	9.0	2.2
Ham & Egg Biscuit	1 serv.	370	19.0	1.1
Ham Egg & Cheese Biscuit	1 serv.	420	23.0	0.8
Regular Roast Beef Sandwich	1 serv.	260	9.0	0.8
Three Pancakes	1 serv.	280	2.0	1.4
KFC				
BBQ Baked Beans	1 serv.	132	2.0	4.0
Biscuit	1 serv.	220	12.0	1.0
Chicken Breast	1 serv	354	23.7	0.0
✔ Corn on the Cob	1 serv.	222	12.0	8.0
Cornbread	1 serv.	175	6.4	0.7
Crispy Fries	1 serv.	210	11.0	3.0
Garden Rice	1 serv.	75	1.0	1.0
Garden Salad	1 serv.	16	0.0	1.0
Green Beans	1 serv.	36	1.0	2.0
Macaroni & Cheese	1 serv.	162	8.0	0.0
Macaroni Salad	1 serv.	248	17.0	1.0
Mashed Potatoes & Gravy	1 serv.	70	1.0	2.0
Mean Greens	1 serv.	52	2.0	3.0
Pasta Salad	1 serv.	135	8.0	1.0
Potato Salad	1 serv.	180	11.0	2.0
Potato Wedges	1 serv.	192	9.0	3.0
Red Beans & Rice	1 serv.	114	3.0	3.0
Vegetable Medley Salad	1 serv.	126	4.0	3.0
LONG JOHN SILVER				
Catfish Fillet	1 serv.	860	42.0	0.1
Chicken, Light Herb	1 serv.	120	4.0	0.0
Fish/Lemon, Entree	1 serv.	570	12.0	2.0
Fish & More Entree	1 serv.	890	48.0	1.7
Fish Sandwich Platter	1 serv.	870	38.0	4.1
Garden Salad	1 serv.	170	9.0	2.1
Homestyle Fish, 6 Piece	1 serv.	1260	64.0	2.3
Light Fish, Paprika	1 serv.	300	2.0	1.3
Light Fish/Lemon Crumb	1 serv.	270	5.0	2.4

ITEM NAME	PORTION	CAL	FAT	FIBER
✔ Mixed Vegetables	1 serv.	60	2.0	5.9
Seafood Platter	1 serv.	970	46.0	5.3
Seafood Salad	1 serv.	270	7.0	1.3
Seafood Salad, Scoop	1 serv.	210	5.0	0.6
Shrimp Scampi	1 serv.	610	18.0	0.0

McDONALD'S

ITEM NAME	PORTION	CAL	FAT	FIBER
Bacon Bits	1 pkg.	15	1.0	0.0
Bacon, Egg & Cheese Biscuit	1 serv.	450	27.0	1.0
Barbecue Sauce	1 pkg.	50	0.0	0.0
Biscuit with Spread	1 serv.	260	13.0	1.0
Cheeseburger, Quarter Pounder	1 item	520	29.0	2.0
Cheeseburger	1 item	320	13.0	2.0
Chicken McNuggets	6 pieces	300	18.0	0.0
Cone, Yogurt, Vanilla Lowfat				
Frozen	1 serv.	120	0.5	0.0
Cookies, Chocolaty Chip	1 pkg.	280	14.0	1.0
Cookies, McDonaldland	1 pkg.	260	9.0	1.0
Croutons	1 pkg.	50	1.5	0.0
Danish				
Apple	1 slice	360	16.0	1.0
Cheese	1 serv.	410	22.0	0.0
Cinnamon and Raisin	1 item	430	22.0	1.0
Raspberry	1 item	400	16.0	1.0
Egg McMuffin	1 item	290	13.0	1.0
Eggs, Scrambled	2 eggs	170	12.0	0.0
English Muffin	1 serv.	140	2.0	1.0
Filet O Fish	1 item	360	16.0	1.0
French Fries, Regular	1 serv.	210	10.0	2.0
✔ Large	1 serv.	450	22.0	5.0
✔ Super Size	1 serv.	540	26.0	6.0
Hamburger	1 item	270	9.0	2.0
Big Mac	1 item	510	26.0	3.0
McLean Deluxe	1 item	340	12.0	2.0
Quarter Pounder	1 item	420	20.0	2.0
Hashbrown Potato	1 serv.	130	8.0	1.0
Honey Sauce	1 pkg.	45	0.0	0.0
Hot Cakes with Syrup & Margarine	1 serv.	560	14.0	2.0
Hot Mustard Sauce	1 pkg.	60	3.5	1.0
McChicken Sandwich	1 serv.	490	29.0	2.0
McGrilled Chicken Classic	1 serv.	250	3.0	2.0
Milk Shake				
Chocolate, Small	1 serv.	350	6.0	1.0
Strawberry, Small	1 serv.	340	5.0	0.0
Vanilla, Small	1 serv.	310	5.0	0.0

ITEM NAME	PORTION	CAL	FAT	FIBER
Muffin, Apple Bran	1 serv.	180	0.5	1.0
Pie, Apple	1 serv.	290	15.0	1.0
Pork Sausage	1 serv.	170	16.0	0.0
Salad				
Chef	1 serv.	210	11.0	3.0
Chunky Chicken	1 serv.	160	5.0	3.0
Garden	1 serv.	80	4.0	3.0
Side	1 serv.	45	2.0	2.0
Salad Dressing, Red French				
Reduced Calorie	1 pkg.	160	8.0	1.0
Salad Dressing, Thousand Island	1 pkg.	190	13.0	1.0
Sausage Biscuit	1 item	430	29.0	1.0
Sausage McMuffin with Egg	1 item	440	29.0	1.0
Sundae, Yogurt				
Hot Caramel Lowfat	1 serv.	310	3.0	1.0
Hot Fudge Lowfat	1 serv.	290	5.0	2.0
Strawberry Lowfat Frozen	1 serv.	240	1.0	1.0
Sweet and Sour Sauce	1 pkg.	60	0.2	0.0

SUBWAY

ITEM NAME	PORTION	CAL	FAT	FIBER
✔ BMT Sandwich on Honey Wheat Roll	1 item	1011	57.0	6.0
✔ BMT Sandwich on Italian Roll	1 item	982	55.0	5.0
✔ Club Sandwich on Honey Wheat	1 item	722	23.0	6.0
✔ Club Sandwich on Italian Roll	1 item	693	22.0	5.0
✔ Cold Cut Combo Sandwich on Italian	1 item	853	40.0	5.0
✔ Cold Cut Combo Sandwich on Wheat	1 item	883	41.0	6.0
✔ Ham & Cheese Sandwich on Italian	1 item	643	18.0	5.0
✔ Ham & Cheese Sandwich on Wheat	1 item	673	2.0	6.0
Meatball Sandwich on Italian Roll	1 item	918	44.0	3.0
✔ Roast Beef Sandwich on Italian Roll	1 item	689	23.0	5.0
✔ Roast Beef Sandwich on Wheat Roll	1 item	717	24.0	6.0
Salad Dressing, Buttermilk Ranch	1 serv.	348	37.0	0.0
Salad Dressing, Lite Italian	1 serv.	23	1.0	0.0
Seafood/Crab Sandwich on Wheat	1 item	1015	58.0	2.5
✔ Spicy Italian Sandwich on Italian	1 item	1043	63.0	5.0
✔ Steak & Cheese Sandwich on Italian	1 item	765	32.0	6.0
✔ Turkey Breast Sandwich on Wheat Roll	1 item	674	20.0	7.0

TACO BELL

ITEM NAME	PORTION	CAL	FAT	FIBER
Burrito				
✔ Bean	1 item	387	14.0	9.5

ITEM NAME	PORTION	CAL	FAT	FIBER
Beef	1 item	431	21.0	2.0
Chili Cheese	1 item	391	18.0	4.8
Combination	1 item	412	16.0	10.1
Double Beef Supreme	1 item	457	22.0	5.7
Supreme	1 item	443	19.0	11.3
✔ Mexican Pizza	1 serv.	575	37.0	5.8
Nachos	1 serv.	346	19.0	1.4
Pintos & Cheese	1 serv.	190	9.0	4.9
Taco, Soft	1 item	228	12.0	3.8
Taco, Regular	1 item	183	11.0	2.4
Taco Bell Grande	1 item	355	23.0	4.5
Taco Salad				
✔ No Salsa, No Shell	1 serv.	502	31.0	7.0
✔ with Salsa, No Shell	1 serv.	520	31.0	7.0
✔ with Salsa, Shell	1 serv.	941	61.0	7.9
✔ Tostada, Regular	1 item	243	11.0	8.4
✔ Tostada, Beefy	1 item	334	17.0	5.2

WENDY'S

ITEM NAME	PORTION	CAL	FAT	FIBER
✔ Baked Potato Plain	1 serv.	250	0.0	5.0
✔ with Bacon & Cheese	1 serv.	510	17.0	9.9
✔ with Broccoli & Cheese	1 serv.	500	25.0	5.0
with Cheese	1 serv.	550	24.0	3.6
✔ with Chili and Cheese	1 serv.	510	20.0	8.0
✔ with Sour Cream & Chives	1 serv.	460	24.0	5.0
Cheese Tortellini/Spaghetti Sauce	1 serv.	120	1.0	1.0
Cheeseburger, Single with Everything	1 serv.	490	27.0	2.7
Chicken Club Sandwich	1 serv.	520	25.0	2.3
Chicken Salad	1 serv.	35	3.0	0.2
✔ Chili, Small	1 serv.	190	6.0	6.0
French Fries, Regular Size	1 serv.	360	17.0	4.6
Hamburger, Plain	1 item	350	15.0	2.8
Double	1 serv.	540	27.0	2.3
Kids Meal	1 serv.	270	9.0	1.3
Quarter Pound Big Classic	1 serv.	480	23.0	2.3
Single with Everything	1 serv.	440	23.0	2.7
Refried Beans	1 serv.	70	2.0	3.0
Spanish Rice	1 serv.	70	1.0	0.7
✔ Taco Salad with Taco Chips	1 serv.	660	37.0	10.5
Tuna Salad	1 serv.	100	6.0	0.3

FATS & OILS

Pure fats and oils are fiber-free. You can, however, find small amounts of fiber in unrefined oils that contain small amounts of seed materials left after pressing.

ITEM NAME	PORTION	CAL	FAT	FIBER
Beef Tallow	1 tbsp.	126	14.0	0.0
Butter, Regular or Sweet, Pat	1 item	36	4.0	0.0
Cooking, Spray, Olive Oil Flavor - Pam	1 serv.	2	1.0	0.0
Flax Seed Oil, Unfiltered, High Lignan, Organic - Barleans	1 tbsp.	115	14.0	1.0
Ghee	1 oz.	250	28.0	0.0
Margarine, Veg Oil	1 cup	784	88.0	0.0
Mayonnaise - Kraft	1 tbsp.	100	12.0	0.0
Molly Mcbutter	1 serv.	8	0.0	0.0
Oil, All types	1 tbsp.	126	14.0	0.0
Shortening, (Partially Hydrogenated Vegetable Oil)	1 tbsp.	126	14.0	0.0

FROZEN FOODS

Frozen foods are a mixed bag when it comes to fiber. Look for entrees that are based on high-fiber components, such as legumes, vegetables, and grains.

ITEM NAME	PORTION	CAL	FAT	FIBER
MEAT-BASED ENTREES				
✔ Beef BrocFiberi Beijing - Healthy Choice	1 pkg.	330	3.0	5.0
Beef Burgundy - Light and Elegant Dinner	1 item	230	4.0	1.6
✔ Beef Chop Suey & Rice - Stouffer's	1 serv.	300	9.0	5.2
Beef Dinner - Swanson Frozen Dinner	1 item	320	9.0	3.3
✔ Beef Enchilada Dinner - Healthy Choice	1 pkg.	410	8.0	9.0
✔ Beef Mesquite Barbecue Sauce - Healthy Choice	1 pkg.	310	4.0	6.0
Beef Pepper Oriental, Frozen - La Choy	1 cup	216	4.5	0.1
Beef Pepper Steak, Rice - Ultra Slim Fast	1 item	310	5.0	1.8

ITEM NAME	PORTION	CAL	FAT	FIBER
Beef Pie - Stouffer's	1 serv.	500	32.0	2.9
Beef & Pork Cannelloni - Lean Cuisine	1 serv.	260	10.0	2.3
✔ Beef Pot Pie, Hungry Man - Swanson	1 pkg.	620	29.0	6.0
✔ Beef Pot Roast, Light & Healthy - Budget Gourmet	1 item	210	8.0	7.0
✔ Beef Sirloin, Wine Sauce - Light & Healthy	1 item	230	6.0	6.0
Beef Stroganoff - Budget Gourmet Light	1 item	290	12.0	1.3
Beef Stroganoff, Noodles - Stouffer's	1 serv.	390	20.0	1.8
Beef Teriyaki, Rice/Vegetables - Stouffer's	1 serv.	290	8.0	1.5
Beef Tips Francais - Healthy Choice	1 pkg	280	5.0	4.0
Beef Tortellini - Stouffer's	1 serv.	360	12.0	2.3
✔ Burrito, Beef & Bean - El Monterey	1 item	270	11.0	8.0
Cabbage - Stuffed with Meat - Lean Cuisine	1 serv.	220	10.0	3.8
Chili Con Carne with Beans - Stouffer's	1 serv.	260	10.0	4.7
Ham - Banquet Frozen Dinner	1 item	369	12.2	2.6
Lasagna, Meat with Sauce - Lean Cuisine	1 serv.	270	8.0	3.5
Lasagna/Meat Sauce - Budget Gourmet Light	1 item	300	13.0	3.2
Manicotti, Cheese/meat - Budget Gourmet	1 serv.	450	26.0	2.4
✔ Meatloaf - Banquet Frozen Dinner	1 item	412	23.7	5.4
✔ Meatloaf Dinner - Healthy Choice	1 pkg.	320	8.0	7.0
✔ Mexican Dinner - Swanson Frozen Dinner	1 item	590	29.0	6.7
Oriental Beef - Lean Cuisine	1 pkg.	250	8.0	4.0
Pork, Sweet & Sour, Frozen - La Choy	1 cup	378	14.1	0.3
✔ Salisbury Steak Banquet Frozen Dinner	1 item	390	24.6	5.3
✔ Healthy Choice	1 pkg.	260	6.0	5.0
with Gravy - Stouffer's	1 serv.	250	14.0	3.7
Sausage/Egg/Cheese Biscuit - Swanson	1 item	490	30.0	3.0
Sausage/French Toast, Great Starts - Swanson	1 pkg.	410	26.0	3.0

ITEM NAME	PORTION	CAL	FAT	FIBER
Sirloin Salisbury Steak - Budget Light	1 item	260	13.0	3.2
✔ Sirloin Salisbury Steak - Light & Healthy	1 item	260	9.0	6.0
✔ Sirloin Tips/Noodles, Hungry Man - Swanson	1 pkg.	450	16.0	9.0
Sirloin Tip/Vegetables - Budget Gourmet	1 serv.	310	18.0	2.6
Spaghetti				
Beef/Mushroom - Ultra Slim Fast	1 item	370	9.0	4.6
Meat Sauce - Healthy Choice	1 item	310	6.0	3.9
Meat Sauce - Weight Watchers	1 pkg.	250	6.0	6.0
✔ Veal Parmigiana Dinner - Swanson	1 pkg.	400	18.0	5.0
✔ Veal Steak - Classic Lite Frozen Dinner	1 item	280	8.0	5.8
✔ Yankee Pot Roast Dinner - Healthy Choice	1 item	280	5.0	5.0

POULTRY-BASED ENTREES

ITEM NAME	PORTION	CAL	FAT	FIBER
Chicken, French, with Vegetables - Budget Light	1 item	240	9.0	4.2
Chicken, Fried, Dinner, Dark Meat - Swanson	1 pkg.	560	28.0	4.0
Chicken, Grilled, with Salsa - Lean Cuisine	1 pkg.	240	6.0	4.0
✔ Chicken, Herbed, Breast meat - Light and Healthy	1 item	240	7.0	6.0
Chicken, Mandarin - Budget Gourmet Light	1 pkg.	250	5.0	4.0
Chicken, Scalloped - Stouffer's	1 serv.	420	25.0	4.3
✔ Chicken, Southwestern - Healthy Choice	1 pkg.	300	3.0	6.0
Chicken, Sweet and Sour - Budget Gourmet	1 serv.	350	7.0	1.7
Chicken, Turkey, BrocFiberi, Cheese - Lean Pockets	1 item	260	8.0	4.0
Chicken a l'Orange, Almonds - Lean Cuisine	1 serv.	260	5.0	3.6
✔ Chicken Breast Parmesan - Lean Cuisine	1 pkg.	220	5.0	5.0
Chicken Carbonara - Lean Cuisine	1 pkg.	290	8.0	4.0
Chicken Cashew with Rice - Stouffer's	1 serv.	380	16.0	1.6
Chicken Chow Mein - Lean Cuisine	1 pkg.	210	5.0	2.0

ITEM NAME	PORTION	CAL	FAT	FIBER
✔ Chicken Dinner - Swanson Frozen	1 item	660	33.0	6.2
✔ Chicken Enchiladas Suiza - Healthy Choice	1 pkg.	270	4.0	5.0
✔ Chicken Fettucini - Ultra Slim Fast	1 item	400	10.0	6.5
✔ Chicken Fiesta - Weight Watchers	1 pkg.	220	4.0	6.0
✔ Chicken Florentine - Le Menu Frozen Dinner	1 item	510	28.0	6.7
Chicken Imperial - Healthy Choice	1 item	230	4.0	3.0
Chicken Kiev - Le Menu Frozen Dinner	1 item	500	30.0	4.4
✔ Chicken Mesquite - Con Agra Frozen Dinner	1 serv.	340	1.0	5.7
Chicken Pasta Shells - Stouffer's	1 item	400	22.0	3.0
Chicken Pie - Stouffer's	1 serv.	530	33.0	3.3
Chicken Pot Pie, Hungry Man - Swanson	1 pkg.	650	35.0	3.0
Chicken Vegetable Marsala - Lean Cuisine	1 pkg.	220	1.0	3.0
✔ Chicken Vegetable Rotini - Ultra Slim Fast	1 item	310	3.0	5.1
Turkey a la King/Rice - Budget Gourmet	1 serv.	390	18.0	2.4
✔ Turkey Breast, Stuffed - Light & Healthy	1 item	230	6.0	8.0
Turkey Dinner - Swanson Frozen Dinner	1 item	340	10.0	3.6
Turkey Gravy Casserole - Stouffer's	1 serv.	360	17.0	1.9
Turkey Mushrooms - Healthy Choice	1 pkg.	220	4.0	3.0
✔ Turkey Pot Pie, Hungry Man - Swanson	1 pkg.	650	34.0	5.0
✔ BrocFiberi & Cheese Baked				

CHEESE ENTREES

ITEM NAME	PORTION	CAL	FAT	FIBER
Potato - Weight Watchers	1 pkg.	230	7.0	6.0
✔ Cheddar BrocFiberi & Potatoes - Healthy Choice	1 pkg.	310	5.0	8.8
✔ Cheese Ravioli Parmigiana - Healthy Choice	1 pkg.	250	4.0	6.0
Cheese Lasagna/Vegetable - Budget Light	1 item	290	9.0	4.8
Cheese Tortellini, Tomato Sauce - Stouffer's	1 serv.	360	16.0	2.5
✔ Enchiladas, Cheese - Stouffer's	1 serv.	590	40.0	7.8
Macaroni & Cheese - Healthy Choice	1 pkg.	290	5.0	4.0

ITEM NAME	PORTION	CAL	FAT	FIBER
Quiche, Classic French, Individual - Nancy's	1 pkg.	520	37.0	1.0
Vegetable, 3 Cheese - Kraft Pasta & Cheese	1 cup	360	16.0	3.7

PIZZA

ITEM NAME	PORTION	CAL	FAT	FIBER
Cheese				
Crisp & Tasty - Jenos	1 serv.	270	14.0	2.1
Lean Cuisine	1 serv.	310	10.0	2.9
Microwave - Pillsbury	1 serv.	240	10.0	2.0
Party - Totinos	1 serv.	340	17.0	2.7
Combination				
Microwave - Pillsbury	1 serv.	310	15.0	2.3
Party - Totinos	1 serv.	380	21.0	2.7
French Bread				
Cheese - Lean Cuisine	1 item	330	7.0	4.0
Cheese - Stouffer's	1 item	340	13.0	2.9
Deluxe - Lean Cuisine	1 item	330	6.0	5.0
Hamburger - Stouffer's	1 serv.	410	19.0	1.2
Pepperoni - Lean Cuisine	1 item	330	7.0	4.0
Pepperoni/Mushroom - Stouffer's	1 serv.	430	22.0	3.2
Vegetable Deluxe - Stouffer's	1 serv.	420	20.0	4.7
Golden Topping - Fox Deluxe	1 serv.	240	11.0	1.5
Hamburger, Party - Totinos	1 serv.	370	19.0	1.0
Party Pizza - Totino's	½ pie	380	21.0	2.0
Pepperoni - Lean Cuisine	1 serv.	330	7.0	4.0
Pepperoni - Red Baron	⅕ pie	360	19.0	2.0
Sausage - Stouffer's	1 serv.	360	18.0	2.3
Sausage, Party - Totinos	1 serv.	390	21.0	2.6
Sausage & Pepperoni - Tombstone	⅕ pie	340	18.0	2.0
✔ Spicy Chicken - Wolfgang Puck	½ pie	360	16.0	5.0
Supreme				
Light - Tombstone	1 serv.	261	9.0	2.4
Supreme Single, Thin - Tombstone	1 serv.	308	18.0	2.6
Super - Tombstone	⅙ pie	350	18.0	2.0
Vegetable, Light - Tombstone	⅕ pie	240	7.0	3.0
Vegetable, Party - Totinos	1 serv.	300	13.0	3.1
Pizza Rolls - Jenos	1 serv.	250	13.0	1.6

PASTA DISHES

ITEM NAME	PORTION	CAL	FAT	FIBER
Angel Hair Marinara - Weight Watchers	1 pkg.	170	2.0	4.0
✔ Fettucini Alfredo - Linda McCartney's	1 pkg.	520	18.0	5.0
✔ Fettucini Alfredo - Weight Watchers	1 pkg.	220	6.0	6.0

39

ITEM NAME	PORTION	CAL	FAT	FIBER
Fettucini Primavera - Lean Cuisine	1 pkg.	260	8.0	4.0
Fiesta Lasagna - Stouffer's	1 serv.	430	22.0	3.5
✔ Garden Lasagna - Weight Watchers	1 pkg.	230	7.0	6.0
Lasagna, Vegetable - Stouffer's	1 serv.	420	24.0	4.8
Linguini, Shrimp/Tomato - Healthy Choice	1 item	230	2.0	3.5
✔ Pasta, Oriental - Stouffer's	1 serv.	300	14.0	10.9
✔ Pasta & Garden Vegetable - Light Balance	1 item	190	1.0	5.4
✔ Pasta Penne with Sun Dried Tomatoes - Weight Watchers	1 pkg.	290	9.0	8.0
Pasta Primavera - Ultra Slim Fast	1 item	340	9.0	4.2
Rigatoni Pomodoro Italiano - Michelina's	1 pkg.	290	8.0	4.0
✔ Vegetable Lasagna - Le Menu Frozen Dinner	1 item	400	24.0	5.1
Zucchini Lasagna - Lean Cuisine	1 pkg.	240	4.0	4.0

SEAFOOD & OTHERS

ITEM NAME	PORTION	CAL	FAT	FIBER
Breakfast Burrito with Eggs, Hot & Spicy - Swanson	1 item	220	7.0	3.0
Deviled Crab - Mrs. Pauls	1 item	180	9.0	1.0
Egg Roll, Vegetable, Large, Frozen - La Choy	1 item	150	7.1	0.7
Fish and Chips - Van De Kamps Dinner	1 item	500	30.0	4.7
Scrambled Eggs/Bacon/Potatoes, Great Starts - Swanson	1 pkg.	290	19.0	1.0
Shrimp Marinara - Ultra Slim Fast	1 item	290	3.0	4.6
✔ Tuna Noodle Casserole - Weight Watchers	1 pkg.	240	7.0	5.0

VEGETARIAN ENTREES

ITEM NAME	PORTION	CAL	FAT	FIBER
Beef Style Meatless 3/8" Slices - Worthington	1 slice	110	7.0	3.0
Better'n Burgers, Meatless - Morningstar	1 pattie	70	0.0	3.0
Better'n Eggs, Meatless - Morningstar	1/4 cup	20	0.0	0.0
Bolono - Worthington	3 slices	80	3.5	2.0
Breakfast Links, Meatless - Morningstar	2 links	90	5.0	2.0
Breakfast Strips, Meatless - Morningstar	2 strips	60	5.0	0.5

ITEM NAME	PORTION	CAL	FAT	FIBER
Chicken, Sliced, Meatless - Worthington	2 slices	80	4.5	0.5
Chic, Ketts ⅜" Slices - Worthington	2 slices	120	7.0	2.0
✔ Chik Nuggets - Loma Linda	5 pieces	240	16.0	5.0
Chik Patties - Morningstar	1 item	170	10.0	2.0
Corn Dogs, Meatless - Loma Linda	1 item	200	9.0	3.0
Corned Beef, Sliced, Meatless - Worthington	4 slices	140	9.0	2.0
Cream of Spinach - Stouffer's	1 serv.	210	15.0	3.2
Crispychik Patties - Worthington	1 patty	170	9.0	4.0
Deli Franks, Meatless - Morningstar	1 link	110	7.0	2.0
Diced Chik, Meatless - Worthington	¼ cup	80	4.5	0.5
Dinner Entree, Meatless - Natural Touch	1 pattie	220	15.0	2.0
Dinner Roast, ¾" Slices, Meatless - Worthington	1 slice	180	12.0	3.0
Fillets, Meatless - Worthington	2 pieces	180	10.0	4.0
Fried Chik'n - Loma Linda	1 piece	180	15.0	0.7
Fripats - Worthington	1 pattie	130	6.0	3.0
Garden Grain Pattie - Natural Touch	1 pattie	160	7.0	2.0
Garden Vege Patties - Morningstar	1 pattie	110	4.0	4.0
Gnocchi, Potato Dumplings, Raw - Bernardi	1 oz.	60	0.0	0.3
✔ Golden Croquettes - Worthington	4 pieces	210	10.0	6.0
Griddle Steaks - Loma Linda	1 piece	130	7.0	4.0
Grillers, Meatless - Morningstar	1 pattie	140	7.0	3.0
Ground Meatless Vegetarian Beef - Worthington	½ cup	80	2.5	3.0
Ground Meatless Vegetarian Sausage - Worthington	½ cup	110	6.0	3.0
Leanies - Worthington	1 link	110	8.0	1.0
Lentil Rice Loaf, 1" Slices - Natural Touch	1 slice	170	9.0	4.0
Links, Breakfast, Frozen - Morningstar	1 item	45	2.5	1.0
✔ Nine Bean Loaf, 1" Slices - Natural Touch	1 slice	160	8.0	5.0
Okara Patty - Natural Touch	1 pattie	160	12.0	3.0
Pea Pods, Snow, Frozen - La Choy	1 cup	48	0.2	4.2
✔ Potato Slices/Vegetables/ Cream Sauce - Healthy Choice	1 pkg.	200	4.0	6.0
Prime Patties - Morningstar	1 pattie	130	5.0	3.0
Prosage Links - Worthington	2 links	120	9.0	2.0

ITEM NAME	PORTION	CAL	FAT	FIBER
Prosage Roll, ⅝" Slice - Worthington	1 slice	140	10.0	2.0
Ratatouille - Stouffers Frozen Side Dish	1 item	60	3.0	2.3
Salami, Meatless - Worthington	3 slices	130	8.0	2.0
Scalloped Potatoes - Kraft	1 serv.	140	5.0	2.3
Scramblers - Morningstar	1 cup	140	0.0	0.0
✔ Sizzle Burger - Loma Linda	1 pattie	200	12.0	6.0
Smoked Beef Slices, Meatless - Worthington	6 slices	120	6.0	3.0
Smoked Turkey Slices, Meatless - Worthington	3 slices	140	10.0	2.0
Stakelets, Meatless - Worthington	1 piece	140	8.0	2.0
Stir Fry Vegetables, Frozen - La Choy	1 cup	47	0.3	0.3
Stripples, Meatless - Worthington	2 strips	60	5.0	0.0
✔ Three Bean Chili - Lean Cuisine	1 pkg.	210	6.0	7.0
Tuno, Drained, Meatless - Worthington	½ cup	80	6.0	1.0
✔ Veelets - Worthington	1 pattie	180	9.0	5.0
Vege Burger - Natural Touch	1 pattie	140	6.0	4.0
Vege Frank - Natural Touch	1 link	45	6.0	2.0
✔ Vegetarian Beef Pie - Worthington	1 pie	410	24.0	6.0
✔ Vegetarian Chicken Pie - Worthington	1 pie	450	27.0	8.0
✔ Vegetarian Chili - Right Course	1 serv.	280	7.0	10.2
Vegetarian Egg Rolls - Worthington	1 roll	180	8.0	2.0
✔ Vegetarian Harvest Burger - Green Giant	1 item	140	4.0	5.0
Wham, Meatless - Worthington	2 slices	80	5.0	0.0
Whole Wheat Pancakes, Lite Links - Swanson	1 oz.	64	2.9	1.1
✔ Zucchini Lasagna - Healthy Choice	1 pkg.	330	1.5	11.0

FRUITS

High in vitamins and minerals and low in fat, fruits are also a natural when it comes to fiber. Dried fruits, such as figs, dates, apricots, and prunes, are packed with fiber, as are all the different types of berries. All things considered, the fruit category offers the most flavorful way to add fiber to your diet. A word of caution, though, about fruit roll-type snack foods. Check the list and read product labels carefully, since many are actually fiber-poor fabricated foods that include only small amounts of real fruit.

ITEM NAME	PORTION	CAL	FAT	FIBER

FRESH, FROZEN, & DRIED FRUITS

ITEM NAME	PORTION	CAL	FAT	FIBER
Acerola, Raw	1 cup	31	0.3	1.1
Apple, unpeeled	1 med.	80	1.0	4.0
✔ Apples, Dried, Uncooked	1 cup	209	0.3	8.6
Apricot, Raw, Without Pit	1 item	17	0.1	0.7
Apricots				
✔ Dried, Cooked, Sugar Added	1 cup	305	0.4	8.3
✔ Dried, Sulfured, Uncooked	1 cup	309	0.6	10.1
Frozen, Sweetened	1 cup	237	0.2	4.1
Avocado, Raw, Florida	¼ med.	85	6.8	2.1
Avocado, Raw, California	¼ med.	77	7.5	1.7
Avocado Pear (Apokat)	1 oz.	51	5.4	1.6
Banana, Fresh	1 item	110	0.5	4.0
Banana Flakes, Dehydrated or				
Powdered	1 tbps.	22	0.1	0.5
✔ Blackberries, Fresh	1 cup	75	0.6	8.9
✔ Blackberries, Frozen, Unsweetened	1 cup	97	0.6	7.6
Blueberries				
✔ Dried - Trader Joe's	½ cup	320	0.0	10.0
Fresh	1 cup	81	0.6	3.9
Frozen, Unsweetened	1 cup	79	1.0	5.0
✔ Boysenberries, Frozen,				
Unsweetened	1 cup	66	0.4	5.2
✔ Breadfruit, Fresh	¼ med.	99	0.2	11.7
Cantaloupe	¼ med.	50	0.0	0.9
Carambola (Star Fruit), Fresh	1 item	42	0.4	1.5
Casaba Melon, Fresh	1 cup	44	0.2	2.0
✔ Cherimoya, Fresh	1 item	514	2.2	13.0
Cherries				
Montmorency, Dried -				
Trader Joe's	½ cup	240	0.8	3.0
Sour, Fresh	1 cup	77	0.5	1.9
Sweet	21 items	90	1.0	3.0
Sweet, Frozen, Sweetened	1 cup	231	0.3	8.7
Coconut, Dried, Shredded	1 cup	466	33.0	3.9
✔ Cranberries, Dried - Pilgrim Joe's	½ cup	180	0.5	5.0
Cranberries, Fresh	1 cup	54	0.2	4.6
Currants				
European Black, Fresh	1 cup	71	0.5	4.8
Zante, Dried - S&W	½ cup	260	0.0	4.0
Date	1 item	24	0.0	0.7
✔ Elderberries, Fresh	1 cup	106	0.7	12.3
Figs				
Dried, Uncooked	1 cup	507	2.3	18.5
Fresh	1 item	37	0.2	3.2

ITEM NAME	PORTION	CAL	FAT	FIBER
Kadota - S&W	5 items	140	1.0	3.0
Gooseberries, Fresh	1 cup	66	0.9	4.0
✔ Grapefruit	½ med.	70	0.5	5.0
Grapefruit, Red/Pink/White, Fresh	1 cup	74	0.2	3.2
Grapes	1½ cups	90	1.0	1.0
Groundcherries, Fresh	1 cup	80	1.1	4.2
✔ Guava, Common, Fresh	1 med.	46	0.5	5.4
✔ Guava, Strawberry, Fresh	1 med.	65	0.6	6.4
Honeydew Melon	⅒ med.	50	0.0	1.0
Jackfruit, Fresh	1 cup	83	0.3	0.9
Kiwifruit	2 med.	100	1.5	4.0
Kumquat, Fresh	2 med.	12	0.0	1.3
Lemon, Fresh, Without Peel	1 item	17	0.2	0.6
Lime, Fresh	1 med.	20	0.0	3.0
✔ Loganberries, Frozen	1 cup	81	0.5	7.1
Lychee, Canned, Drained	1 oz.	21	0.1	0.1
Lychee, Dried	1 avg.	8	0.0	0.1
Mango, Fresh	1 item	135	0.6	4.8
Melon, Casaba	⅙ melon	74	0.7	1.5
Melon Balls, Cantaloupe or				
Honeydew, Frozen	1 cup	57	0.4	2.6
Mixed Fruit, Frozen, Sweetened	1 cup	245	0.5	3.0
Mulberries, Fresh	1 cup	60	0.5	2.4
Nectarine, Fresh	1 item	67	0.6	1.6
Oheloberries, Fresh	1 cup	39	0.3	3.6
Olive, Ripe, Canned, Large	1 item	5	0.5	0.1
✔ Orange	1 med.	80	0.0	5.0
Orange Peel, Fresh	1 tbsp.	6	0.0	0.2
✔ Papaya, Fresh	1 med.	247	0.6	8.3
Passion Fruit, Purple, Fresh	1 item	18	0.1	2.2
Peach	1 med.	40	0.0	2.0
✔ Peaches, Dried	1 cup	382	1.2	14.0
✔ Peaches, Frozen, Sliced,				
Sweetened	1 cup	235	0.3	6.0
Pear	1 med.	100	1.0	4.0
Pears				
✔ Dried	1 cup	472	1.1	13.8
Fresh, Asian	1 med.	57	0.3	4.4
Fresh, Bartlett, with Skin	1 med.	98	0.7	4.7
Persimmons, Japanese, Dried	1 item	93	0.2	0.6
Persimmons, Native, Fresh	1 item	32	0.1	0.4
Pineapple				
3" diameter, ¾" thick slices	2 slices	70	0.0	1.0
Fresh, Diced	1 cup	76	0.7	1.9
✔ Frozen, Sweetened	1 cup	208	0.3	5.4
Plantains, Cooked	1 cup	179	0.3	3.5

ITEM NAME	PORTION	CAL	FAT	FIBER
Plantains, Fresh	1 item	218	0.7	4.1
Plum, Fresh, Prune Type	1 item	20	0.0	0.6
Plum, Fresh, Japanese & Hybrid	1 item	36	0.4	1.4
Plums	2 med.	80	1.0	2.0
Pomegranate, Fresh	1 item	105	0.5	1.1
✔ Pricklypears, Fresh	1 item	42	0.5	5.6
✔ Prunes, Dried	1 cup	385	0.8	11.0
✔ Prunes, Dried, Cooked, Without Sugar	1 cup	227	0.5	7.5
Pummelo, Sections, Fresh	1 cup	72	0.1	1.9
Quinces, Fresh	1 item	52	0.1	1.8
Raisins				
Golden Seedless - S&W	½ cup	260	0.0	4.0
✔ Seeded	1 cup	488	0.9	8.7
✔ Seedless	1 cup	435	0.7	6.1
Thompson Seedless - S&W	½ cup	260	0.0	4.0
✔ Raspberries, Fresh	1 cup	261	0.7	9.1
✔ Raspberries, Frozen, Sweetened	1 cup	258	0.4	11.0
Rhubarb				
Cooked from Frozen, Added Sugar	1 cup	278	0.1	4.8
✔ Cooked from Raw, Added Sugar	1 cup	380	0.0	5.4
Fresh	1 cup	26	0.2	2.2
Salmonberries, Alaska	1 cup	44	0.1	1.0
Strawberries				
✔ Dried - Trader Joe's	1 cup	280	0.0	6.0
Fresh	8 med.	70	0.5	3.0
✔ Frozen, Sweetened, Whole	1 cup	199	0.4	5.6
Tamarinds, Fresh	1 item	5.0	0.0	0.1
Tangerines	1 med.	80	1.0	3.0
Watermelon	1/18 med.	90	0.0	1.0

CANNED FRUITS

ITEM NAME	PORTION	CAL	FAT	FIBER
Apple Butter	1 tbsp.	37	0.2	0.2
Apples, Spiced Apple Rings - S&W	2 items	25	0.0	1.0
✔ Apples, Sweet, Heated	1 cup	137	0.9	5.1
Applesauce				
Gravenstein, Unsweetened - S&W	1 cup	100	0.0	4.0
Sweetened	1 cup	194	0.5	3.1
Unsweetened	1 cup	105	0.1	3.7
Apricots, Light Syrup Pack	1 cup	159	0.1	4.6
Apricots Water Pack	1 cup	66	0.4	4.1
✔ Blackberries, Heavy Syrup Pack	1 cup	236	0.4	17.7
Blueberries, Heavy Syrup Pack	1 cup	255	0.9	2.8

45

ITEM NAME	PORTION	CAL	FAT	FIBER
✔ Blueberries, Wild Maine, Heavy Syrup - S&W	1 cup	140	0.0	12.0
✔ Boysenberries, Heavy Syrup Pack	1 cup	225	0.3	5.7
Cherries				
Pitted, Royal Anne - S&W	1 cup	280	0.0	2.0
Sour, Red, Light Syrup	1 cup	189	0.2	2.3
Sour, Red, Water Pack	1 cup	88	0.2	2.2
Sweet, Light Syrup Pack	1 cup	170	0.4	1.8
Sweet, Water Pack	1 cup	114	0.3	0.6
Crab Apples, Spiced - S&W	1 item	35	0.0	1.0
Cranberry Sauce, Sweetened	1 cup	418	0.4	3.2
Cranberry, Whole, Sauce, Sweetened - S&W	1 cup	400	0.0	4.0
✔ Figs, Heavy Syrup Pack	1 cup	228	0.3	8.9
✔ Figs, Water Pack	1 cup	131	0.2	5.2
Fruit Cocktail, Light Syrup Pack	1 cup	145	0.2	2.8
✔ Gooseberries, Heavy Syrup Pack	1 cup	184	0.5	7.0
Grapefruit, Juice Pack	1 cup	92	0.2	1.6
Grapes, Thompson, Water Pack	1 cup	98	0.3	1.7
✔ Mixed Fruit, Chunky, Natural Style - S&W	1 cup	140	0.0	6.0
Oranges, Mandarin, Light Syrup - S&W	1 cup	133	0.0	1.3
Peaches				
Cling, Sliced, Juice Pack - S&W	1 cup	160	0.0	2.0
Halves/Slices, Light Syrup	1 cup	136	0.1	2.5
Pears				
Extra Light Syrup Pack	1 cup	116	0.3	4.2
Juice Pack - S&W	1 cup	160	0.0	4.0
Halved, in Water, Dietetic	½ item	16	0.0	0.7
Pineapple				
Bits, Water Pack	1 cup	79	0.2	2.0
Juice Pack	1 cup	150	0.2	1.8
Sliced, Dietetic, Water	1 slice	47	0.0	1.8
Plums, Purple, Light Syrup	1 cup	158	0.3	2.5
Plums, Whole Purple - S&W	1 cup	260	0.0	4.0
✔ Prunes, Heavy Syrup Pack	1 cup	246	0.5	8.6
Prunes, Stewed, Heavy Syrup - S&W	8 items	210	0.0	4.0
✔ Raspberries, Heavy Syrup Pack	1 cup	234	0.3	6.5
Strawberries, Heavy Syrup Pack	1 cup	234	0.7	3.1
Tangerines				
Juice Pack	1 cup	92	0.1	1.5
Light Syrup Pack	1 cup	154	0.3	1.4
Mandarins, Juice Pack	1 cup	92	0.1	0.9
Mandarins, Light Syrup	1 cup	154	0.3	0.9

ITEM NAME	PORTION	CAL	FAT	FIBER

FRUIT & FRUIT-FLAVORED PRODUCTS

ITEM NAME	PORTION	CAL	FAT	FIBER
Bugs Bunny Fruit-Flavored Snacks - Betty Crocker	1 pouch	90	1.0	0.0
Fruit Bar				
Fat Free Apple - Health Valley	1 item	140	1.0	3.7
Fat Free Apricot - Health Valley	1 item	140	1.0	3.7
Fat Free Date - Health Valley	1 item	140	2.0	4.0
Fat Free Raisin - Health Valley	1 item	140	1.0	3.7
Oat Bran Jumbo - Health Valley	1 item	140	2.0	4.0
Rice Bran Jumbo - Health Valley	1 item	160	5.0	3.7
Fruit-by-the-Foot - Betty Crocker	1 roll	80	1.5	0.0
Fruit Leather Bars	1 item	81	1.2	0.5
Fruit Leather Pieces	1 serv.	92	1.9	0.6
Fruit Leather Rollups	1 item	73	0.6	0.5
Fruit Rollups - Betty Crocker	1 roll	55	0.8	0.0
Fruit String Thing - Betty Crocker	1 pouch	80	1.0	0.0
Gushers Fruit Flavored Snacks	1 pouch	90	1.0	0.0
Real Fruit, Asst. Flavors - Barbara's	1 bar	50	0.0	0.0
Tazmanian Devil Fruit Flavored Snacks - Betty Crocker	1 pouch	90	1.0	0.0
X-Men Fun Snacks - Betty Crocker	1 pouch	90	1.0	0.0

GRAINS

Grains come from the seeds of plants, and just about every grain seed is surrounded by an outer layer, or bran, that nature designs to protect the seed. This bran layer is our single best food source of insoluble fiber.

Foods such as whole wheat flour include the entire grain, so they are naturally high in fiber. Contrast this with the lower-fiber "white" wheat flour, where the bran is not used. The fiber content of pasta follows the same theme, with whole grain pastas being significantly higher in dietary fiber.

If you're looking for a quick and convenient way to increase the fiber in your diet, consider adding small quantities of fiber-rich pure brans, such as oat, wheat, rice, or corn bran, to sauces, baked goods, cereals, or other foods.

ITEM NAME	PORTION	CAL	FAT	FIBER

FLOURS

ITEM NAME	PORTION	CAL	FAT	FIBER
✔ Amaranth - Arrowhead Mills	1 cup	440	6.0	8.0

ITEM NAME	PORTION	CAL	FAT	FIBER
✔ Arrowroot	1 cup	457	0.1	5.1
✔ Barley	1 cup	401	1.9	20.2
✔ Buckwheat - Whole Groat	1 cup	402	3.7	16.9
✔ Corn, Masa, Sifted	1 cup	416	4.3	6.5
✔ Corn, Whole Grain	1 cup	422	4.5	18.0
Cottonseed	1 cup	498	9.2	2.8
Lima Bean	1 cup	377	1.5	2.2
✔ Millet - Arrowhead Mills	1 cup	440	4.0	8.0
✔ Oat - Arrowhead Mills	1 cup	360	6.0	12.0
Peanut, Defatted	1 cup	223	5.5	1.6
Potato	1 cup	628	1.3	2.6
✔ Quinoa - Ancient Harvest	1 cup	528	8.0	9.2
Rice, White	1 cup	578	2.2	3.0
✔ Rice, Brown	1 cup	574	4.4	5.5
Rye, Light	1 cup	374	1.4	3.7
Rye, Dark	1 cup	415	3.4	4.0
✔ Sesame, Lowfat	1 cup	333	1.8	6.0
Soy, Defatted	1 cup	364	1.2	2.7
✔ Soy, Lowfat	1 cup	313	5.9	7.0
✔ Spelt - Arrowhead Mills	1 cup	400	2.0	20.0
Sunflower Seed, Partially Defatted	1 cup	441	4.4	6.0
✔ Triticale, Whole Grain	1 cup	439	2.4	7.1
Wheat, White				
All Purpose - Gold Medal	1 cup	400	0.0	2.0
Bread - Gold Medal	1 cup	400	2.0	2.0
Cake/Pastry - Enriched	1 cup	395	0.9	2.6
Hygluten - Supreme	1 cup	400	0.0	3.0
Tortilla Mix	1 cup	450	11.8	3.4
Self Rising - Gold Medal	1 cup	400	0.0	2.0
✔ Wheat, Whole Wheat Blend - Gold Medal	1 cup	400	2.0	8.0
✔ Wheat, Whole Wheat - Gold Medal/Robin Hood	1 cup	360	2.0	12.0

GRAINS

ITEM NAME	PORTION	CAL	FAT	FIBER
100% Organic Amaranth - Health Valley	1 oz.	85	0.5	4.4
✔ Barley, Pearled, Light, Cooked	1 cup	193	0.7	8.9
Buckwheat Groats, Roasted, Cooked	1 cup	182	1.2	4.0
✔ Bulgur, Cooked	1 cup	152	0.4	6.8
✔ Corn Bran, Crude	1 cup	170	0.7	13.0
✔ Corn Grits, Dry Mix	1 cup	579	1.8	18.6
Cornmeal				
✔ Degermed, Enriched, Dry	1 cup	505	2.3	7.2

ITEM NAME	PORTION	CAL	FAT	FIBER
✔ Whole Grain, Dry	1 cup	442	4.4	18.8
Cornstarch	1 cup	488	0.1	1.2
Couscous, Near East, Prepared from Mix	1 cup	190	0.5	2.0
Croutons, Herb Seasoned	1 cup	100	0.0	1.4
✔ Millet, Cooked	1 cup	286	2.4	11.4
✔ Millet, Raw	1 cup	756	8.5	29.2
✔ Oat Bran, Raw	1 cup	231	6.6	12.5
Oat Bran Shake, Toasted - Pride O the Farm	1 tsp.	17	0.0	1.0
✔ Oats, Whole Grain, Uncooked	1 cup	607	10.8	20.8
✔ Quinoa, Whole or Ground	1 cup	636	9.9	8.8
Rice, Brown				
Long Grain, Cooked	1 cup	216	1.8	3.3
Medium Grain, Cooked	1 cup	218	1.6	3.3
Uncle Ben's	1 cup	220	1.8	2.1
Rice, Fried	1 cup	204	1.1	1.0
Rice, White				
Glutinous, Cooked	1 cup	234	0.5	2.4
Long Grain, Enriched, Cooked - Uncle Ben's	1 cup	160	0.0	<1.0
Medium Grain, Enriched, Raw	1 cup	600	0.0	4.0
Rice, Wild, Cooked	1 cup	166	0.6	2.6
Rice, Wild & Long Grain, Raw - Hinode	1 cup	680	2.0	4.0
✔ Rice Bran - Crude	1 cup	262	17.3	8.2
✔ Rice Polished	1 cup	278	13.4	7.4
✔ Rye, Whole, Dry	1 cup	566	4.2	8.9
Shake 'N Bake				
Italian Herb - General Foods	1 pkg.	320	4.0	0.0
Original Chicken - General Foods	1 pkg.	320	8.0	0.0
Tangy Honey Chicken - General Foods	1 pkg.	360	8.0	0.0
✔ Sorghum, Whole, Dry	1 cup	651	6.3	28.6
Soy Meal, Defatted, Raw	1 cup	149	2.9	0.7
Waffle/Pancake Mix, Dry	1 cup	431	2.2	4.0
Wheat				
✔ Durum	1 cup	651	4.7	10.3
✔ Hard Red, Spring	1 cup	632	3.7	9.8
✔ Hard Red, Winter	1 cup	628	3.0	10.3
✔ Hard White	1 cup	657	3.3	6.6
✔ Soft White	1 cup	571	3.3	5.7
✔ Soft Red, Winter	1 cup	556	2.6	9.4
Sprouted	1 cup	214	1.4	3.4
✔ Wheat Bran, Crude	1 cup	130	2.6	7.7

ITEM NAME	PORTION	CAL	FAT	FIBER
✔ Wheat Germ, Crude	1 cup	414	11.2	11.9
Wheat Germ, Toasted, Kretchmer	2 tbsp.	50	1.0	2.0

PASTA

Listed values are for one cup of prepared pasta.

ITEM NAME	PORTION	CAL	FAT	FIBER
Fettuccine, Fresh - Contadina	1 cup	200	2.8	1.6
Fettuccine, Fresh, Spinach-Contadina	1 cup	216	3.2	3.2
✔ Lasagna, Whole Wheat, Wheat Germ - Health Valley	1 cup	170	1.0	7.2
Linguine, Fresh - Contadina	1 cup	192	2.4	1.6
Macaroni	1 cup	197	0.9	2.2
DeCecco	1 cup	400	2.0	4.0
Protein	1 cup	189	0.2	3.3
Spirals, Vegetable	1 cup	172	0.1	5.8
Vegetable	1 cup	172	0.1	2.7
Whole Wheat	1 cup	174	0.8	2.8
Noodles				
Cellophane/Long Rice	1 cup	491	0.1	0.0
Chow Mein, Canned - La Choy	1 cup	300	16.0	1.7
Egg, Enriched, Cooked	1 cup	213	2.4	2.7
✔ Egg, Spinach, Enriched	1 cup	211	2.5	6.4
Ramen, Oriental	1 cup	207	8.6	2.0
Rice, Canned - La Choy	1 cup	260	8.0	1.1
Soba, Buckwheat	1 cup	190	0.6	1.0
Somen, Wheat	1 cup	202	0.4	1.0
Wheat	1 cup	65	3.6	0.2
Quinoa, Cooked - Ancient Harvest	1 cup	180	2.0	2.5
Rotini Select - Pritikin	1 cup	190	1.0	4.8
Soba Noodles, Japanese, Cooked	1 cup	113	0.1	2.5
Somen Noodles, Japanese, Cooked	1 cup	230	0.3	3.9
Spaghetti				
100% Organic - Health Valley	1 oz.	85	0.5	3.6
Enriched, Cooked	1 cup	197	0.9	2.1
Protein Fortified, Cooked	1 cup	229	0.3	1.1
✔ Spinach, Organic - Health Valley	1 cup	170	1.0	7.2
✔ Whole Wheat	1 cup	180	1.0	6.6
✔ Spelt, Cooked - VitaSpelt	1 cup	190	1.5	5.0

NUTS & SEEDS

Nuts and seeds have fibrous outer coats when growing to protect them from the elements and allow them to remain viable until they can sprout into a new plant.

These coats are the main reason that nuts and seeds are a good source of fiber. They can provide a fiber boost at snack time, or be used as an ingredient in cooking and baking.

ITEM NAME	PORTION	CAL	FAT	FIBER
Almond Butter, Plain	1 tbsp.	101	9.5	1.8
Almonds				
Asst. Varieties, 25 nuts -				
Blue Diamond	1 oz.	150	14.0	2.5
Unsalted	1 cup	910	76.5	4.3
Beechnuts, Dried	1 oz.	164	14.2	2.6
Brazil, Dried, Shelled	1 oz.	186	18.8	2.2
✔ Breadfruit Seeds, Roasted	1 oz.	59	0.8	8.0
Butternuts, Dried	1 oz.	174	16.2	2.4
Cashew Butter, Salt Added - Marantha	1 tbsp.	105	8.0	3.0
Cashews, Roasted/Salted,				
18 nuts - Planters	1 oz.	170	14.0	1.0
Chestnuts				
Chinese, Dried	1 oz.	103	0.5	2.2
Chinese, Fresh	1 oz.	64	0.3	2.2
Roasted	1 oz.	68	0.3	2.2
Coconut, Dried, Flaked, Canned	½ cup	170	12.2	2.2
Coconut, Shredded, Premium -				
Bakers	1 serv.	135	9.0	1.3
Coconut Flesh, Mature	1 oz.	101	9.8	1.3
✔ Filberts/Hazelnuts, Roasted, Salted	½ cup	477	45.8	6.1
Flax Seed, Linseed	1 oz.	141	9.6	4.8
Hazelnuts, Oregon	1 oz.	166	17.0	3.9
Hickory, Dried	1 oz.	187	18.3	2.4
Macadamia, Oil Roasted,				
12 nuts - Mauna Loa	1 oz.	200	21.0	3.0
Mixed, Roasted/Salted, 20 nuts -				
Planters	1 oz.	200	18.0	2.0
Peanut Butter, Natural Creamy -				
Health Valley	1 tbsp.	85	7.0	1.3
Peanuts				
Honey Roasted, 35 nuts - Eagle	1 oz.	180	14.0	2.0
Roasted, 35 nuts	1 oz.	166	14.0	2.0
Spanish, Roasted/Salted,				
53 nuts - Planters	1 oz.	180	14.0	2.0
Pecans, Roasted	1 oz.	195	20.2	2.2
Pistachios, Natural/Red, 22 nuts -				
Trader Joe's	1 oz	170	12.0	3.0
Pumpkin/Squash Seeds, -				
Roasted, Salted	1 oz.	148	12.0	3.9

ITEM NAME	PORTION	CAL	FAT	FIBER
Sesame Butter (Tahini) - Westbrae Organic	2 tbsp.	200	17.0	3.0
✔ Sesame Seed, Roasted, Whole	1 oz.	161	13.6	5.3
✔ Soybean Kernels, Roasted	1 cup	489	25.9	9.2
Sunflower Kernels, Roasted	½ cup	385	33.5	4.6
Walnut, Black/Persian/English	½ cup	380	35.3	2.4
Watermelon Seeds, Dried	1 oz.	150	12.2	4.1

SAUCES, GRAVIES, & DRESSINGS

Sauces, gravies, and dressings are not typically high in fiber. They may provide small amounts if vegetables are included, or if fiber-based thickeners are used to stiffen the texture of the finished product.

ITEM NAME	PORTION	CAL	FAT	FIBER
GRAVY				
Au Jus, Dehydrated, Prepared	1 cup	32	1.3	2.5
Beef, Canned	1 cup	13	55.0	0.1
Chicken, Dehydrated, Prepared	1 cup	83	2.0	2.7
Mushroom, Canned	1 cup	119	6.5	1.0
Mushroom - Franco-American	1 cup	80	4.0	0.8
Turkey - Franco-American	1 cup	100	4.0	0.8
SAUCES				
Barbecue, Ready to Serve	1 cup	188	4.5	2.3
Bearnaise, Dehydrated	1 serv.	362	9.0	0.1
Catsup, Tomato, Regular	2 tbsp.	30	0.0	0.5
✔ Chili - Hunt's	1 serv.	117	0.2	5.9
Curry, Dry Mix, Made with Milk	1 cup	269	14.7	0.9
Enchilada - Rosarita	1 oz.	6	0.0	0.3
Mushroom, Dry Mix, Made with Milk	1 cup	227	10.3	0.5
Peanut - House of Tsang	1 tbsp.	45	2.5	0.7
Pepper, Habanero, Kiss of Fire - Calido Chile Traders	1 tbsp.	20	1.0	1.0
Peppers, Hot Chili, Red, Canned, Sauce	1 cup	51	1.5	4.7
Pizza - Ragu	1 cup	120	4.0	4.0
Plum, Canned - La Choy	1 tbsp.	20	0.0	0.1
Soy	1 tbsp.	10	0.0	0.0
Spaghetti				
✔ Bombolina - Newman's Own	1 cup	200	10.0	14.0

ITEM NAME	PORTION	CAL	FAT	FIBER
✔ Chunky Garden - Ragu	1 cup	240	8.0	6.0
Garlic-Herb & ExChunky - Healthy Choice	1 cup	100	1.0	4.0
✔ Mushroom - Newman's Own	1 cup	120	4.0	6.0
Sun-Dried Tomato - Classico	1 cup	160	9.0	4.0
✔ Sweet Peppers & Onions - Classico	1 cup	140	8.0	6.0
Traditional - Prego	1 cup	300	12.0	4.0
Stroganoff, Mix, Prepared	1 cup	272	10.7	1.2
Sweet & Sour, Dehydrated	1 serv.	389	0.1	0.1
Taco, Green - LaVictoria	1 tbsp.	0.0	0.0	0.5
Taco, Red - LaVictoria	1 tbsp.	5.0	0.0	0.5
Tartar	1 tbsp.	106	11.6	0.1
Teriyaki, Dehydrated	1 serv.	283	2.0	0.1
Tomato, Canned	1 cup	74	0.4	3.4
Tomato, Italian Recipe - S&W	1 cup	70	0.0	4.0
White, Thick	1 cup	495	39.0	1.0

OTHER DRESSINGS

ITEM NAME	PORTION	CAL	FAT	FIBER
Cheese, Cheddar, All Natural - Kraft	1 tbsp.	60	4.0	0.0
✔ Guava, Sauce, Cooked	1 cup	86	0.3	6.8
Horseradish, Prepared	1 tbsp.	6	0.0	0.3
Jelly, Asst. Flavors	1 tsp.	6	0.0	0.0
Mustard, Dijon - Grey Poupon	1 tsp.	5	0.0	0.1
Mustard, Yellow, Prepared	1 tsp.	5	0.1	0.1
Pickle Relish				
Cut or Chopped, Sour	1 cup	27	1.3	2.7
Cut or Chopped, Sweet	1 cup	193	0.8	2.7
Dill - Vlasic	1 tbsp.	5	0.0	0.5
Salad Dressing				
Blue Cheese	1 tbsp.	77	8.0	0.1
French	1 tbsp.	67	6.4	0.1
Italian	1 tbsp.	69	7.1	0.1
Russian, Low Calorie	1 tbsp.	23	0.7	0.2
Sesame Seed	1 tbsp.	68	6.9	0.2
Sweet and Sour	1 tbsp.	29	0.3	0.3
Thousand Island	1 tbsp.	59	5.6	0.6
Salsa				
Chile, Green Tomatillo - Rosarita	2 tbsp.	10	0.0	0.5
Medium - Rosarita	2 tbsp.	10	0.0	0.5
S&W	1/4 cup	20	0.0	1.0
Thick & Chunky - Pace	2 tbsp.	10	0.0	1.0

SNACK FOODS & CHIPS

Snack foods are usually based on grains such as corn and wheat, and as such, they have some fiber potential. It's the exception rather than the rule, though, because most are made from bran-less flours. As you scan the list, you'll find that there are a few chips and pretzels that offer 3 to 4 grams of fiber per serving.

When making selections from this group, note the fat content since many snack foods and chips are deep-fat fried. When examining the tables as well as product labels, always make note of the number of chips used to calculate the nutritional information.

ITEM NAME	PORTION	CAL	FAT	FIBER
CORN CHIPS				
Amazing Bakes - Barbara's	24 chips	100	1.0	1.0
Barbecue	1 oz	148	9.3	1.3
Blue Corn, Organically Grown - Barbara's	15 chips	140	7.0	1.0
Cones, Plain	1 oz.	145	7.6	1.9
Cones, Nacho Cheese	1 oz.	152	9.0	1.3
Doritos				
Cool Ranch	1 serv.	140	7.0	1.8
Nacho Cheese, Light	1 serv.	110	4.0	1.1
Toasted Corn, Light	1 serv.	150	7.0	1.9
Fritos - Wild Mild Ranch	1 serv.	150	9.0	1.3
Hooplas, Original - Keebler	1 serv.	140	8.0	1.3
Terra Vegetable Chips	1 serv.	140	7.0	3.0
POPCORN				
Butter, Full Fat, Singles - Pop Secret	1 cup	35	2.2	0.7
Butter Flavor				
Pop Secret	1 cup	35	2.0	0.5
Light - Pop Secret	1 cup	25	1.0	0.5
Light, Singles - Pop Secret	1 cup	25	1.2	0.7
Buttery Burst - Pop Secret	1 cup	35	2.0	0.5
Buttery Burst, Light - Pop Secret	1 cup	25	1.0	0.5
Caramel, Fat Free - Louise's	1 cup	100	0.0	1.0
Caramel with Peanuts	1 cup	171	3.3	2.6
Cheese Flavor	1 cup	58	3.7	1.1
Honey Caramel Keebler	1 serv.	120	3.0	1.7
Natural Flavor				
Pop Secret	1 cup	35	2.0	0.5
Light - Pop Secret	1 cup	25	1.0	0.5
Light, Singles - Pop Secret	1 cup	25	1.2	0.7

ITEM NAME	PORTION	CAL	FAT	FIBER
Oil & Salt, Popped	1 cup	41	2.0	0.7
Plain, Popped	1 cup	40	0.5	0.8
Popcorn Cakes	1 item	38	0.3	1.5
Popcorn Cakes, Cheddar - Chico San	1 item	50	2.0	0.4
White Cheddar - Keebler	1 cup	70	5.0	2.8

POTATO CHIPS

Barbecue - Barbara's	1¼ cup	160	10.0	1.0
Cheese Flavor	1 oz.	140	7.7	1.4
Light - Kettle	1 oz.	142	7.3	1.4
No Salt - Barbara's	1¼ cup	150	10.0	1.0
Plain - Kettle	1 oz.	158	10.9	1.4
Ripple - Barbara's	1¼ cup	150	10.0	1.0
Salted, Lays	18 chips	150	10.0	1.0
Light - Ruffles	1 serv.	120	6.0	1.2
Sour Cream and Onion	1 oz.	150	9.6	0.3

TORTILLA CHIPS

Baked - Guiltless Gourmet	22 chips	110	1.0	4.0
Baked - Tostitos	13 chips	110	1.0	2.0
Black Bean - Garden of Eatin'	1 serv.	150	7.0	1.0
Thins - Doritos	9 items	140	7.0	1.0
Nacho Cheese - Doritos	11 chips	140	7.0	1.0
Oven Roasted - Smart Temptations	11 chips	110	1.0	1.0
Plain, 100% White corn - Santitas	6 items	140	6.0	1.0
Restaurant Style - Tostitos	6 items	130	6.0	1.0
Tortilla Strips, Salsa Flavor - Laura Scudder's	7 items	140	7.0	1.0

SNACK BARS

Breakfast Bar, Strawberry - Health Valley	1 item	110	0.0	3.0
Cereal Bar, Fat-Free, asst. fruit fillings	1 item	110	0.0	2.0
Chocolate bar, Diet - Figurines	1 item	100	5.0	0.2
Cocoa Almond Crunch Bar - Ultra Slim Fast	1 item	110	4.0	3.0
Cocoa Raspberry Crunch - Ultra Slim Fast	1 item	100	3.0	3.0
Date Bar, from Mix - Betty Crocker	1/12 pkg.	160	7.0	1.0
Fruit Bar, Oat Bran, Nuts - Health Valley	1 bar	150	4.0	2.9

ITEM NAME	PORTION	CAL	FAT	FIBER
Granola Bar				
Carob Chip - Barbara's	1 bar	80	2.0	3.0
Chocolate, Low Fat - Nature Valley	1 bar	110	2.0	1.0
Chocolate Chips - Nature Valley	1 bar	110	4.5	1.0
Chocolate Coated	1 bar	132	7.1	1.0
with Chocolate Marshmallows	1 bar	121	4.4	1.0
Cinnamon & Oats - Barbara's	1 bar	80	2.0	3.0
Date, Fat Free - Health Valley	1 bar	140	1.0	3.7
Oat Bran - Nature Valley	1 bar	110	4.0	1.5
Oats 'N Honey - Barbara's	1 bar	80	2.0	2.0
Oats & Honey, Low Fat - Nature Valley	1 pouch	120	2.0	2.0
Peanut Butter - Barbara's	1 bar	80	3.0	2.0
Peanut Butter - Nature Valley	1 bar	120	6.0	1.0
Plain	1 bar	115	4.9	1.0
with Raisins	1 bar	127	5.0	0.9
Strawberry - Health Valley	1 bar	140	0.0	3.0
Variety Pack - Betty Crocker	1 bar	105	4.0	1.0
Granola Bites, Blueberry, Fat Free - Health Valley	1 bar	140	1.0	3.7
Granola Bites, Raspberry, Fat Free - Health Valley	1 item	140	1.0	3.7
Granola Clusters - Nature Valley	1 item	150	3.0	1.7
✔ Peanut Butter Bar - Slim Fast	1 item	140	6.0	7.0
Pop Tarts	1 cup	713	23.5	1.5
Snack Bar, Assorted Flavors - Health Valley	1 item	100	3.0	2.8
Vanilla Bar - Figurines	1 item	100	6.0	0.2

OTHER SNACKS

ITEM NAME	PORTION	CAL	FAT	FIBER
Apples, Fried - Luck's	1 cup	260	0.0	4.0
Cheese Balls - Planters	1 cup	128	8.0	0.8
Cheetos - Lite Cheese Flavored Snack Chips	1 serv.	120	6.0	1.1
Combos - Cheddar Pretzel	1 item	14	0.6	0.1
Corn Cakes	1 item	35	0.2	1.3
✔ Corn Kernels, Whole Grain	1 cup	606	7.9	18.5
Pinta (Pinto Bean) Chips, Regular - Barbara's	13 chips	130	6.0	2.0
Pretzels				
Bavarian - Barbara's	2 items	100	1.5	3.0
Honeysweet - Barbara's	2 items	100	1.0	3.0
Mini - Barbara's	18 items	100	1.5	4.0
Mr. Salty Pretzel Sticks - Nabisco	88 items	110	0.0	1.0

ITEM NAME	PORTION	CAL	FAT	FIBER
Super Soft - J & J Snack Foods	1 item	193	0.0	1.2
Tiny Twists - Laura Scudder's	20 items	110	0.0	1.0
Puffs				
Apple Cinnamon Caramel Corn - Health Valley	1 cup	110	0.0	2.0
Caramel Corn, Original - Health Valley	1 cup	110	0.0	2.0
Cheese Flavor, Fat Free - Health Valley	1 cup	73	0.0	1.3
Cheese Flavor/Green Onion - Health Valley	1 cup	73	0.0	1.3
Cheese Flavor/Chili, Fat Free - Health Valley	1 cup	73	0.0	1.3
Rice Cakes	1 item	35	0.3	0.2
Brown	1 item	35	0.3	0.2
Brown, Corn	1 item	35	0.3	1.3
Brown, Sesame Seed	1 item	35	0.3	0.2
Low Sodium	1 item	35	0.2	0.2
Sandwich Cracker Snacks (see Breads)				
Sesame Sticks	35 pieces	110	2.5	4.0
Shoestring Potatoes Pik-Nik - S&W	1 cup	240	14.7	1.3
Snack Mix - Pepperidge Farm	1 serv.	140	8.0	1.0
Sun Chips, Original - Frito Lay	1 serv.	140	7.0	1.9
Sweet Potato Chips - Barbara's	1 cup	140	8.0	2.0
Taro Chips - Ray's	1 cup	120	6.0	4.0

SOUPS

Because of their versatility, soups are a convenient way to add fiber to your diet. Note how soups based on legumes, such as peas, beans, and lentils, or vegetables, such as broccoli, quickly turn a soup into a high-fiber dish—some varieties have over 10 grams per cup. As with other foods, keep an eye on the grams of fat per serving.

ITEM NAME	PORTION	CAL	FAT	FIBER
Listed values are for one cup of soup prepared according to directions.				
Asparagus	1 cup	173	8.2	0.6
Bean				
Black	1 cup	235	3.4	4.6
Spicy with Couscous, Dry - Health Valley	1/3 cup	130	0.0	5.0
Turtle	1 cup	218	0.7	4.3

ITEM NAME	PORTION	CAL	FAT	FIBER
Turtle, Boiled	1 cup	241	0.6	3.3
✔ Vegetable, Fat Free - Health Valley	1 cup	110	0.0	12.0
Zesty with Rice - Health Valley	⅓ cup	100	0.0	4.0
✔ Bean, Five Vegetable, Chunky - Health Valley	1 cup	140	0.0	13.0
✔ Bean, Navy, Dry - Knorr	1 pkg.	140	0.0	5.0
✔ Bean with Bacon	1 cup	347	11.9	9.2
Beef, Country Vegetable, Chunky, Single Serv - Campbells	1 can	200	5.0	4.0
Beef, Oriental Ramen - Maruchan	½ pkg.	190	8.0	1.0
Beef, Sirloin/Country Vegetable, Chunky - Campbell's	1 cup	190	9.0	4.0
Beef Noodle	1 cup	84	3.1	1.5
Broccoli, Cream of, Healthy Request - Campbell's	1 cup	140	4.0	2.0
✔ Broccoli Carotene Soup, Super - Health Valley	1 cup	70	0.0	7.0
Broth, Scotch	1 cup	161	5.3	1.2
Celery, Cream of - Campbell's	1 cup	220	14.0	2.0
Cheese	1 cup	155	10.5	2.0
Cheese, Prepared with Milk	1 cup	230	14.6	2.0
Chicken, Country Vegetable - Campbell's	1 cup	150	4.0	1.6
Chicken, Cream of - Campbell's	1 cup	260	16.0	2.0
Chicken, Cream of	1 cup	233	14.7	0.5
Chicken Alphabet - Campbell's	1 cup	160	2.0	2.0
Chicken Chunky, Ready to Eat	1 cup	178	6.6	0.8
Chicken Corn Chowder, Chunky Soup - Campbell's	1 cup	250	15.0	4.0
Chicken and Dumplings, with Milk	1 cup	96	5.5	0.7
Chicken Gumbo - Campbell's	1 cup	120	3.0	2.0
✔ Chicken Minestrone, Tuscany Style, Home - Campbell's	1 cup	160	7.0	5.0
Chicken Noodle	1 cup	150	4.6	1.5
Chunky Soup - Campbell's	1 cup	130	4.0	2.0
Healthy Request - Campbell's	1 cup	160	3.0	2.0
Chicken Oriental Ramen - Maruchan	½ pkg.	190	8.0	1.0
Chicken Pasta - Pritikin	1 cup	100	1.0	1.0
Chicken Pasta & Beans, Dry - Lipton	1 cup	110	1.5	3.0
Chicken Rice				
Chunky Soup - Campbell's	1 cup	130	4.0	2.0
Healthy Choice	1 cup	100	3.0	3.0
Healthy Cookin' - Campbell's	1 cup	120	4.0	1.0

ITEM NAME	PORTION	CAL	FAT	FIBER
Pritikin	1 cup	80	1.0	2.0
Chicken Vegetable	1 cup	149	5.7	1.5
✔ Chili, Three Bean - Pritikin	1 cup	180	1.0	10.0
✔ Chili Beef	1 cup	339	13.2	10.0
Clam Chowder				
Manhattan - Progresso	1 cup	110	2.0	3.0
New England - Healthy Choice	1 cup	140	1.0	7.0
Corn Chowder	1 cup	153	2.7	1.8
Corn Chowder with Tomatoes - Health Valley	½ cup	90	0.0	3.0
✔ Corn & Vegetable, Country, Fat Free - Health Valley	1 cup	70	0.0	7.0
Fiesta Nacho Cheese - Campbell's	1 cup	280	16.0	4.0
French Onion - Campbell's	1 cup	140	5.0	2.0
Garlic & Pasta, Healthy Classics - Progresso	1 cup	100	1.5	3.0
Lentil - Nile Spice	1 pkg.	180	1.5	3.0
✔ Lentil - Pritikin	1 cup	130	<1.0	8.0
✔ Lentil & Carrot, Fat Free - Health Valley	1 cup	90	0.0	14.0
✔ Lentil with Couscous - Health Valley	⅓ cup	130	0.0	5.0
Minestrone	1 cup	167	5.0	1.5
Lipton	1 cup	110	2.0	4.0
Fat Free - Health Valley	1 cup	80	0.0	11.0
Pritikin	1 cup	90	1.0	3.0
Mushroom with Beef Stock	1 cup	171	8.1	0.6
Mushroom, Cream of	1 cup	220	14.0	2.0
Noodle, Chicken Flavored with Vegetables - Health Valley	⅓ cup	100	0.0	4.0
Onion, Dehydrated	1 cup	27	0.6	0.7
Pasta Italiano - Health Valley	½ cup	140	0.0	3.0
Pea, Green	1 cup	165	2.9	4.8
Pepperpot	1 cup	208	9.3	0.5
Pork, Oriental Ramen - Maruchan	½ pkg.	190	8.0	1.0
Potato, Cream of, with Milk	1 cup	148	6.5	0.5
Potato, Creamy with Broccoli - Health Valley	⅓ cup	70	0.0	2.0
Red Beans & Rice - Nile Spice	1 pkg.	190	1.5	3.0
Salmon Broth, King - Alaska	1 cup	4.0	0.2	0.1
Shrimp, Cream of	1 cup	180	10.4	0.3
Split Pea				
Garden, with Carrots - Health Valley	½ cup	130	0.0	2.0
✔ Healthy Classics Progresso	1 cup	180	2.5	5.0
✔ Pritikin	1 cup	140	<1.0	10.0

ITEM NAME	PORTION	CAL	FAT	FIBER
✔ Yellow	1 cup	379	8.8	8.6
Split Pea & Carrot, Fat Free - Health Valley	1 cup	110	0.0	4.0
✔ Split Pea with Ham, Chunky Soup	1 cup	185	4.0	6.0
Steak & Potato, Chunky Soup - Campbell's	1 cup	160	4.0	3.0
✔ Tomato Vegetable, Fat Free - Health Valley	1 cup	80	0.0	5.0
Turkey, Chunky, Ready to Serve	1 cup	135	4.4	2.5
Vegetable				
14 Garden, Fat Free - Health Valley	1 cup	80	0.0	4.0
Campbell's	1 cup	180	2.0	4.0
Hearty - Pritikin	1 cup	90	0.5	3.0
Homestyle, Dry - Mrs. Grass	½ pkg.	70	0.0	2.0
Vegetarian-Pritikin	1 cup	100	0.0	3.0
Vegetable Barley, Fat Free - Health Valley	1 cup	90	0.0	4.0
Vegetable Beef - Campbell's	1 cup	160	4.0	4.0
✔ Vegetable Power Carotene - Health Valley	1 cup	70	0.0	6.0
Vegetable with Pasta, Chunky Soup - Campbell's	1 cup	130	3.0	3.0
Vegetarian	1 cup	144	3.9	2.4

SPICES & FLAVORINGS

There's a high concentration of fiber in spices and condiments, but the small quantities of these flavorful substances that are used in foods make them a minor source in the overall diet.

ITEM NAME	PORTION	CAL	FAT	FIBER
Allspice, Ground	1 tsp.	5	0.2	0.4
Amaranth, Raw	1 oz.	10	0.1	0.4
Anise seed	1 tsp.	7	0.3	0.6
Basil, Ground	1 tsp.	4	0.1	0.2
Bay Leaf, Crumbled	1 tsp.	3	0.1	0.3
Caraway Seed	1 tsp.	7	0.3	0.8
Cardamon, Ground	1 tsp.	6	0.1	0.4
Carob Powder	1 tbsp.	27	0.1	0.4
Celery Seed	1 tsp.	8	0.5	0.2
Chervil, Dried	1 tsp.	1	0.0	0.1
Chili Powder	1 tsp.	8	0.4	0.7
Chives, Fresh	1 tsp.	1	0.0	0.1

ITEM NAME	PORTION	CAL	FAT	FIBER
Cilantro, Fresh	1 serv.	1	0.0	0.8
Cinnamon, Ground	1 tsp.	5	0.1	0.5
Cloves, Ground	1 tsp.	7	0.4	0.2
Cocoa Powder, Low Fat	1 tbsp.	13	0.6	0.4
Cocoa Powder, Processed with Alkali	1 tbsp.	21	1.7	0.3
Coriander Leaf, Dried	1 tsp.	3	0.0	0.1
Coriander Seed	1 tsp.	9	0.5	0.9
Cumin Seeds, Black	1 tsp.	8	0.5	0.3
Cumin Seeds, White	1 tsp.	8	0.5	0.7
Curry Powder	1 tsp.	6	0.3	0.7
Dill Seed	1 tsp.	6	0.3	0.4
Dill Weed, Dried	1 tsp.	3	0.0	0.1
Fennel Seed	1 tsp.	7	0.3	0.3
Fenugreek Seed	1 tsp.	13	0.3	0.4
Garlic Powder	1 tsp.	10	0.0	0.1
Ginger, Ground	1 tsp.	7	0.1	0.1
Ginger, Pickled	1 oz.	27	0.1	0.9
Ginger Root, Crystallized	1 oz.	95	0.1	0.2
Ginger Root, Fresh	1 oz.	15	0.3	0.5
Lemon Grass	1 oz.	17	0.2	0.6
Mace, Ground	1 tsp.	10	0.6	0.1
Marjoram, Dried	1 tsp.	3	0.0	0.2
MSG, Monosodium Glutamate - Accent	1 serv.	0	0.0	0.0
Mustard Dried	1 tsp.	3	0.9	—
Mustard, Prepared Brown	1 tsp.	5	0.3	0.1
Mustard, Prepared Yellow	1 tsp.	4	0.2	0.1
Mustard Seed	1 oz.	143	9.0	0.5
Nutmeg	1 tsp.	11	0.7	0.1
Onion Powder	1 tsp.	7	0.0	0.1
Onions, Dehydrated Flakes	1 tbsp.	16	0.0	0.5
Oregano	1 tsp.	6	0.2	0.3
Paprika	1 tsp.	6	0.3	0.4
Parsley, Dried	1 tsp.	3	0.0	0.1
Parsley, Fresh	1 tbsp.	2	0.0	0.1
Pepper, Red	1 tsp.	6	0.3	0.6
Pepper, White	1 tsp.	6	0.0	0.1
Pepper, Black	1 tsp.	5	0.1	0.5
Poppy Seed	1 tsp.	16	1.3	0.2
Poultry Seasoning	1 tsp.	6	0.2	0.2
Pumpkin Pie Spice	1 tsp.	7	0.3	0.3
Rosemary, Ground	1 tsp.	3	0.2	0.2
Rosemary, Leaves	1 tsp.	4	0.2	0.2
Saffron	1 tsp.	3	0.1	—
Sage, Ground	1 tsp.	3	0.1	0.2

ITEM NAME	PORTION	CAL	FAT	FIBER
Salt, Table	1 tsp.	0	0.0	0.0
Savory, Ground	1 tsp.	3	0.1	0.2
Sesame Seed, Decorticated	1 tsp.	16	1.5	0.3
Tarragon	1 tsp.	3	0.1	0.1
Thyme	1 tsp.	3	0.1	0.2
Tomato, Sun Dried	1 oz.	77	0.1	1.7
Tumeric Root, Dried (Kunyit)	1 oz.	95	1.4	0.9
Tumeric	1 tsp.	7	0.2	—
Yeast, Baker's, Dry, Active	1 tbsp.	34	0.0	3.8
Yeast, Torula	1 tbsp.	33	0.3	3.8

SWEETS, CANDIES, & DESSERTS

Because sweets and candies tend to be chock full of fiber-free sugar, and pastries and desserts tend to be based on fiber-poor white flour, most foods in this category have little fiber to speak of. Choose foods that use peanuts, cocoa (chocolate), or high-fiber fruits, such as figs and raisins.

ITEM NAME	PORTION	CAL	FAT	FIBER
BROWNIES				
Brownie Bites - Hostess	1 item	52	3.0	0.4
Brownie Bites, Walnut - Hostess	1 item	54	3.0	0.4
Double Fudge - Duncan Hines	1/20 pkg.	140	3.0	1.0
Fudge				
Easy Delicious Desserts - Betty Crocker	1/9 pkg.	310	12.0	2.0
Mix - Betty Crocker	1 item	140	2.0	1.0
Mix Robin Hood - Gold Medal	1 item	120	2.0	1.0
Hot Fudge - Pillsbury	1/24 pkg.	130	3.5	<1.0
Dark Chocolate Fudge, Mix - Betty Crocker	1 item	130	2.0	1.0
German Chocolate Supreme - Betty Crocker	1/18 pkg.	160	3.0	1.0
Supreme, Mix - Betty Crocker	1/18 pkg.	140	2.0	1.0
Supreme, with Walnuts, Mix - Betty Crocker	1/18 pkg.	140	4.0	1.0

ITEM NAME	PORTION	CAL	FAT	FIBER
CAKES				
Apple Spice Crumb, Fat Free - Entenmann's	⅛ cake	130	0.0	2.0
Banana, Suzy Q's - Hostess	1 cake	220	10.0	0.5
Banana Crunch - Entenmann's	⅛ cake	220	9.0	<1.0
Banana Crunch, Fat Free - Entenmann's	⅛ cake	140	0.0	2.0
Black Forest Cherry, Bundt, Mix	1 serv.	190	4.0	1.1
Blueberry Crunch, Fat Free - Entenmann's	⅛ cake	140	0.0	2.0
Boston Creme, Supreme - Pepperidge	⅛ cake	260	9.0	0.8
Butter Chocolate, Supermoist - Betty Crocker	1/12 pkg.	190	4.5	1.0
Butter Yellow, Mix, Supermoist	1 serv.	170	2.0	0.3
Butter, Mix - Pillsbury Plus	1 serv.	170	3.0	0.5
Cake, Banana, Mix - Pillsbury Plus	1 serv.	190	4.0	0.4
Carrot				
Entenmann's	⅛ cake	290	16.0	<1.0
Fat Free - Entenmann's	⅛ cake	170	0.0	1.0
Supermoist, Mix	1 serv.	180	3.0	0.5
Cheesecake				
Frozen - Sara Lee	¼ cake	330	12.0	2.0
Frozen - Weight Watchers	1 slice	180	6.0	1.5
New York Style - Jell-O	1 serv.	175	3.0	0.3
Choco-Diles - Hostess	1 cake	210	10.0	1.0
Choco-Licious - Hostess	1 cake	170	6.0	1.0
Chocolate Chocolate Chip, Supermoist Mix	1 serv.	190	5.0	2.1
Chocolate Crunch, Fat Free - Entenmann's	⅛ cake	130	0.0	2.0
Chocolate Free & Light - Sara Lee	1 slice	110	0.0	2.4
Chocolate Fudge				
3-Layer - Pepperidge	⅙ cake	300	16.0	2.0
Entenmann's	⅙ cake	320	15.0	2.0
Supermoist - Betty Crocker	1/12 pkg.	180	4.0	1.0
Chocolate Fudge Iced, Fat Free - Entenmann's	⅙ cake	210	0.0	2.0
Chocolate Loaf, Fat Free - Entenmann's	⅛ loaf	130	0.0	1.0
Chocolate Mousse, Light - Pepperidge	1 item	190	9.0	0.4
Chocolate Pudding, Classic, Mix	1 serv.	220	4.0	0.8
Cinnamon Apple Coffee, Fat Free - Entenmann's	⅛ cake	130	0.0	2.0

ITEM NAME	PORTION	CAL	FAT	FIBER
Cinnamon Streusel Swirl, Mix	1 serv.	200	5.0	0.4
Coconut, 3-Layer - Pepperidge	1/8 cake	300	14.0	1.0
Coffee				
Cinnamon Swirl - Pillsbury	1 slice	180	9.0	0.1
Crumb - Sara Lee	1/8 cake	220	9.0	0.9
Pecan - Sara Lee	1/8 cake	220	12.0	2.0
Creme, Regular - Hostess	1 item	190	5.0	0.3
Crumb - Hostess	1 cake	105	4.0	0.5
Crumb, Light - Hostess	1 cake	75	0.5	0.4
Cupcake				
Chocolate - Hostess	1 cake	170	5.0	1.0
Chocolate Light - Hostess	1 cake	120	1.5	0.8
Devil's Food with Chocolate Icing	1 item	120	4.0	0.7
Orange - Hostess	1 cake	160	5.0	0.8
Dark Chocolate, Mix - Pillsbury Plus	1 serv.	180	5.0	0.8
Devil's Food				
Layer - Pepperidge	1 oz.	111	5.5	0.5
Light, Supermoist - Betty Crocker	1/10 pkg.	210	3.0	2.0
Mix - Microrave Singles	1 item	250	10.0	1.0
Mix - Robin Hood	1/5 cake	190	5.0	1.0
Supermoist - Betty Crocker	1/12 pkg.	180	4.5	1.0
Fruitcake, Dark - Home Recipe	1 slice	57	2.3	0.3
Fudge Marble, Mix - Pillsbury Plus	1 serv.	200	5.0	0.9
Funfetti, Mix - Pillsbury Plus	1 serv.	190	4.0	0.6
German Chocolate, Mix, Supermoist	1 serv.	180	4.0	0.5
German Chocolate - Entenmann's	1/6 cake	320	16.0	0.8
Gingerbread, Mix	1 slice	175	4.0	1.8
Golden, Fudge Iced, Fat Free - Entenmann's	1/6 cake	220	0.0	2.0
Golden, Thick Fudge - Entenmann's	1/6 cake	330	16.0	2.0
Golden, French Crumb, Fat Free - Entenmann's	1/8 cake	140	0.0	2.0
Golden Pound - Classic Dessert, Mix	1 serv.	190	8.0	0.3
Golden Vanilla Mix - Microrave	1 serv.	230	7.0	0.6
Golden Vanilla Mix, Supermoist	1 serv.	180	4.0	0.3
Lemon, Mix, Supermoist	1 serv.	180	4.0	0.2
Lemon Chiffon, Classic Dessert, Mix	1 serv.	190	4.0	0.2
Lemon Pudding, Classic Dessert, Mix	1 serv.	220	4.0	0.5
Marble, Mix, Supermoist	1 serv.	180	4.0	0.8

ITEM NAME	PORTION	CAL	FAT	FIBER
Milk Chocolate, Supermoist - Betty Crocker	1/12 pkg.	180	4.5	1.0
Pound				
All-Butter - Sara Lee	1/4 cake	320	16.0	0.8
Hostess	1/5 cake	350	16.0	1.0
Rainbow Chip, Mix - Supermoist	1 serv.	180	4.0	0.5
Sheet, No Icing - Home Recipe	1 slice	315	12.0	1.0
Sno Balls - Hostess	1 cake	160	5.0	1.0
Sour Cream Chocolate, Supermoist Betty Crocker	1/12 pkg.	190	5.0	1.0
Spice, Mix, Supermoist	1 serv.	180	4.0	0.4
Strawberry, Mix - Pillsbury Plug	1 serv.	180	4.0	0.5
Strawberry Shortcake	1 serv.	344	8.9	2.1
Streusel Type, with Icing, Mix	1 slice	172	7.5	0.9
Sunshine Vanilla, Mix - Pillsbury Plus	1 serv.	180	5.0	0.6
Suzy Q's - Hostess	1 cake	220	9.0	2.0
Tiger Tails - Hostess	1 cake	160	6.0	1.0
Tunnel of Fudge, Bundt, Mix	1 serv.	200	4.0	1.1
Walnut Slice	1 cup	622	46.1	1.2
White - Pillsbury Plus	1 serv.	180	4.0	0.6
White/Chocolate Icing - Home Recipe	1 slice	271	11.0	0.8
Yellow/Chocolate, Mix - Microrave	1 serv.	210	7.0	0.6
Yellow Baseball - Hostess	1 cake	160	3.0	0.0
Yellow, Mix, Supermoist	1 serv.	180	4.0	0.5
Yellow, Mix - Pillsbury Plus	1 serv.	180	5.0	0.6

CANDY BARS

ITEM NAME	PORTION	CAL	FAT	FIBER
100 Grand Bar	1 bar	195	8.5	0.4
Almond Joy	1 pkg.	240	13.0	2.0
Alpine White Chocolate, with Almond	1 bar	349	22.9	0.6
Baby Ruth Chocolate Bar	1 bar	277	13.3	3.3
Bar None Chocolate Bar	1 bar	224	14.6	1.4
Butterfingers Bar	1 bar	266	11.3	2.3
Caramels, Plain/Chocolate	1 oz.	115	3.0	0.8
Coating, Peanut Butter	1 cup	845	50.7	4.9
Cracker Jack - Borden	1 box	150	3.0	1.0
Golden Almond Bar	1 bar	466	32.1	0.9
Golden Three (iii) Bar	1 bar	471	30.0	1.5
Goobers, Chocolate Peanuts	1 piece	51	3.4	0.3
Kit Kat Bar	1 bar	210	11.0	0.6
Krackel Bar	1 bar	371	20.6	1.6
Kudos, Butter Almond	1 bar	180	10.0	0.4

ITEM NAME	PORTION	CAL	FAT	FIBER
M & M				
Almond - Mars	¼ cup	200	12.0	2.0
Peanut - Mars	¼ cup	220	11.0	2.0
Plain - Mars	¼ cup	200	9.0	1.0
Mars Bar	1 bar	233	11.5	0.8
Milky Way Bar	1 bar	260	9.0	0.1
Mounds Bar	1 bar	195	11.7	0.9
Mr Goodbar	1 bar	406	25.5	3.1
Oh Henry Bar	1 bar	246	9.6	1.4
Peanut Bar	1 bar	235	15.2	2.7
Peanut Butter - PB Max	1 bar	240	16.0	1.3
Peanut Butter Cup	1 piece	92	5.4	0.8
Peanut Brittle	1 oz.	123	4.4	0.5
Rolos, Caramel	1 serv.	261	12.0	0.4
Sesame Crunch	1 piece	9	0.6	0.2
Skor Bar	1 bar	211	13.8	0.7
Snickers Bar	1 bar	280	14.0	1.0
Starburst Fruit Chews	1 serv.	234	4.9	0.5
Symphony Bar	1 bar	355	22.0	1.1
Three Musketeers Bar	1 bar	249	7.7	1.0
Toffee, Crunch'n Munch -				
Franklin	1 serv.	160	5.0	1.0
Tootsie Roll	1 oz.	112	2.5	0.3
Twix, Cookie Bar	1 serv.	273	13.4	0.1
Twix, Peanut Butter Cookie Bar	1 serv.	253	14.5	1.2
Whatchamacallit Bar	1 bar	256	13.2	2.0
York Peppermint Patty	1 item	149	3.9	0.2

CHOCOLATE

Bitter, for Baking	1 oz.	145	15.0	4.3
Chips, Semi-Sweet Morsels -				
Nestle's	30 chips	70	4.0	2.0
Chips, Sweet - Germans	1 serv.	200	12.0	2.8
Chocolate, Special Dark Bar	1 bar	376	23.9	5.2
Cocoa, Powder - Nestle's	1 tbsp.	15	1.0	2.0
Cocoa Mix - Nestle's Quick	2 tbsp.	90	0.5	1.0
Fudge, Chocolate, Plain	1 oz.	115	3.0	0.4
Milk Chocolate, with Almonds	1 bar	151	10.1	1.3
Milk Chocolate, with Rice Bar	1 bar	203	10.9	0.9
Milk Chocolate Peanuts	1 cup	773	49.9	4.9
Milk Chocolate Raisins	1 cup	741	28.1	2.9
Semisweet - Bakers	1 square	130	9.0	2.0
Unsweetened - Nestle's	¼ bar	80	7.0	3.0
White, Baking - Nestle's	¼ bar	80	5.0	0.0

ITEM NAME	PORTION	CAL	FAT	FIBER

COOKIES

ITEM NAME	PORTION	CAL	FAT	FIBER
Amaranth -Health Valley	1 item	60	2.0	2.2
Animal Crackers - Sunshine	14 items	140	4.0	<1.0
Apple Cinnamon Oat Bran - Frookie	1 item	45	2.0	1.0
Arrowroot - Nabisco	1 item	20	0.5	<1.0
Chocolate Brownie, Fat Free - Entenmann's	2 items	80	0.0	1.0
Chocolate Chip				
Barbara's	1 item	85	3.5	1.5
Fiber - Keebler	1 item	70	4.0	1.3
Pillsbury	1 item	70	3.0	0.4
from Refrigerated Dough - Nestle	1 item	75	3.0	0.5
Chocolate/Cinnamon - Teddy Graham	1 serv.	70	3.0	0.3
Chocolate Fudge Sandwich - Keebler	1 item	80	4.0	0.4
Chocolate Wafer - Nabisco	1 item	28	0.8	0.2
Fancy Fruit, Assorted - Health Valley	1 item	45	1.5	0.9
Fancy Peanut Chunk - Health Valley	1 item	45	1.5	1.2
Fiber Jumbo - Health Valley	1 item	100	3.0	3.0
Fig - Ultra Slim Fast	1 item	60	0.5	1.0
Fig Bar - Sunshine	1 item	55	1.3	0.5
Fig Bar, Whole Wheat, Fat Free - Mother's	1 item	70	0.0	1.0
Fig Newton - Nabisco	1 item	55	1.3	0.5
Fig Newton, Fat Free - Nabisco	1 item	50	0.0	1.0
Fortune - La Choy	1 item	15	0.1	0.1
French Vanilla Creme - Keebler	1 item	80	4.0	0.1
Fruit Centers, Fat Free, Assorted Flavors - Health Valley	1 item	25	0.3	1.0
Regular - Health Valley	1 item	70	1.0	3.5
Raspberry - Health Valley	1 item	70	0.0	2.0
Jumbo - Health Valley	1 item	70	1.0	3.5
Fruit & Fitness - Health Valley	1 item	100	2.0	2.8
Fruit, Golden				
Apple - Sunshine	1 item	80	1.5	0.5
Cranberry - Sunshine	1 item	70	1.0	0.5
Fruit Jumbo - Health Valley	1 item	70	3.0	1.0
Fruit & Nut - Barbara's	1 item	85	3.5	1.5
Fudge Royals, Mini	15 items	160	8.0	1.0
Ginger Snaps - Sunshine	7 items	130	4.5	0.5

ITEM NAME	PORTION	CAL	FAT	FIBER
Grahams, Fudge Dipped -				
Sunshine	1 item	43	2.3	0.3
Grammy Bears - Sunshine	10 items	140	5.0	1.0
Health Chip - Health Valley	1 item	100	0.0	4.0
Healthy Grahams - Health Valley	1 item	110	3.0	3.0
Honey Jumbo				
Cinnamon - Health Valley	1 item	50	1.5	1.3
Oat Bran - Health Valley	1 item	60	1.5	2.2
Peanut - Health Valley	1 item	70	1.5	0.9
Macaroon	1 item	90	4.5	0.4
Molasses, Iced - Bakery Wagon	1 item	100	2.5	1.0
Oat Bran, Apple, Fiber - Keebler	1 item	70	3.0	1.1
Oat Bran Fruit Jumbos - Health				
Valley	1 item	60	1.5	1.6
Oat Bran Fruit/Nut - Health Valley	1 item	110	4.0	2.8
Oatmeal				
Country Style - Sunshine	3 items	170	7.0	1.0
Fiber Enriched - Keebler	1 item	70	3.0	1.1
Iced - Sunshine	1 item	60	2.5	0.4
Keebler	1 item	80	4.0	0.4
Oatmeal Chocolate Chip,				
Fat Free - Entenmann's	2 items	80	0.0	1.0
Oatmeal Raisin				
Health Valley	1 item	100	0.0	3.0
Pillsbury	1 item	60	2.0	0.4
Original Vanilla - Fiber Classic	1 item	210	8.0	0.1
Peanut Butter				
✔ Fiber Classic	1 item	220	9.0	7.0
Mix	1 item	50	2.6	0.2
Pillsbury	1 item	70	3.0	0.3
Sandwich				
Chocolate - Ultra Slim Fast	3 items	130	3.0	1.0
Choc/Cream - Snackwells	1 item	50	1.3	0.5
Hydrox - Sunshine	1 item	50	2.3	0.3
Hydrox Reduced Fat - Sunshine	1 item	43	1.3	0.3
Oreo - Nabisco	1 item	53	2.3	0.3
Peanut Butter, Nutter Butter				
Bites - Nabisco	10 items	150	7.0	1.0
Vanilla/Creme Filling -				
Snackwells	1 item	55	1.3	0.5
Sugar				
Fiber Enriched - Keebler	1 item	70	3.0	1.1
Old Fashion - Keebler	1 item	80	3.0	0.6
Pillsbury	1 item	70	3.0	0.2
Sugar Wafer/Creme Filling -				
Lady Lee	1 item	40	2.0	0.2

ITEM NAME	PORTION	CAL	FAT	FIBER
Sultana	1 oz.	119	2.4	0.2
Tea Biscuit - Peek Freans	1 item	40	1.3	0.2
Tofu, The Great - Health Valley	1 item	45	1.5	0.7
Vanilla, Dixie - Sunshine	2 items	120	4.5	0.5
Vanilla, Teddy Graham Bearwich	1 serv.	60	2.0	0.2
Vanilla Wafer				
Mother's	1 item	25	1.0	0.1
Nabisco Nilla Wafers	1 item	18	0.6	0.0
Sunshine	1 item	21	1.0	0.1
Vienna Fingers - Sunshine	1 item	70	3.0	0.4
Vienna Fingers, Low Fat -				
Sunshine	1 item	65	1.8	0.4
Wheat - Alphabet	1 oz.	122	2.6	0.1
Wheat-Free, The Great -				
Health Valley	1 item	40	1.5	1.7

DONUTS

ITEM NAME	PORTION	CAL	FAT	FIBER
Bakery - Hostess	1 donut	140	7.0	0.8
Cake				
Devil's Food Crumb	1 donut	175	8.4	1.0
Frosted - Entenmann's	1 donut	400	27.0	1.0
Chocolate Minidonuts - Hostess	3 donuts	132	5.4	0.6
Cinnamon - Hostess	1 donut	110	5.0	0.5
Cinnamon, Low Fat - Entenmann's	1 donut	180	6.0	0.8
Crumb - Hostess	1 donut	130	8.0	0.8
Crumb Gems (Minidonuts) -				
Hostess	3 donuts	160	5.5	0.5
Frosted, Regular - Hostess	1 donut	180	6.0	1.0
Frosted Gems (Minidonuts) -				
Hostess	3 donuts	195	11.5	1.0
Glazed				
Honey Wheat - Hostess	1 donut	250	12.0	1.0
Low Fat - Entenmann's	1 donut	220	6.0	0.8
Mini, Frosted - Entenmann's	2 donuts	270	20.0	1.0
Plain, Old Fashioned - Hostess	1 donut	170	9.0	1.0
Plain, Regular - Hostess	1 donut	120	6.0	0.5
Powdered				
Gems (Minidonuts) - Hostess	3 donuts	175	8.0	0.5
Strawberry Filled Gems				
(Minidonuts) - Hostess	3 donuts	210	9.0	1.0
Rich Chocolate Frosted -				
Entenmann's	1 donut	290	19.0	1.0
Yeast, Glazed	1 donut	205	11.2	1.1

ITEM NAME	PORTION	CAL	FAT	FIBER

FROZEN DESSERTS

ITEM NAME	PORTION	CAL	FAT	FIBER
Frozen Pops, All Types	–	–	–	0.0
Frozen Yogurt, All Types	–	–	–	0.0
Ice Cream Sundae				
Hot Fudge	1 item	297	9.0	1.2
Regular - Dairy Queen	1 item	300	7.0	2.2
Strawberry	1 item	289	8.5	0.7
Ice Cream, Chocolate	1 cup	143	7.3	0.5
Ice Cream Cone, Sugar - Keebler	1 item	45	0.0	0.2
Ice Milk, Vanilla	1 cup	184	5.6	0.0
Ices, Water, All Types	–	–	–	0.0
Pudding Pops				
Chocolate, Frozen	1 item	72	2.2	0.4
Chocolate - Jell-O	1 serv.	79	2.0	0.4
Sherbet, All Types	–	–	–	0.0
Sorbet, All Types	–	–	–	0.0

PIES

ITEM NAME	PORTION	CAL	FAT	FIBER
Apple				
French - Hostess Fruit Pie	1 pie	410	19.0	2.0
Homestyle - Entenmann's	1/6 pie	300	14.0	2.0
Hostess Fruit Pie	1 pie	410	19.0	2.0
Mrs. Smith's	1/6 pie	270	11.0	1.0
Apple Beehive, Fat Free - Entenmann's	1/5 pie	270	0.0	2.0
Banana Cream - Mrs. Smith's	1/4 pie	250	9.0	1.0
Banana Custard, 1 Crust, Baked	1 cup	396	16.6	1.4
Blackberry, 2 Crusts, Baked	1 cup	467	21.1	5.7
Blackberry - Hostess Fruit Pie	1 pie	400	17.0	2.0
Blueberry, 2 Crusts, Baked	1 cup	465	20.7	3.3
Blueberry - Hostess Fruit Pie	1 pie	400	17.0	2.0
Butter Tarts, Baked	1 cup	534	14.6	1.9
Cherry - Hostess Fruit Pie	1 pie	430	19.0	1.0
Cherry Beehive, Fat Free - Entenmann's	1/5 pie	270	0.0	1.0
Cherry Streusel, Free/Light - Sara Lee	1 slice	160	2.0	0.9
Chocolate Meringue, 1 Crust, Baked	1 cup	474	22.6	2.6
Coconut Custard, 1 Crust, Baked	1 cup	421	22.4	2.9
Custard, 1 Crust, Baked	1 cup	390	19.9	0.6
Lemon - Hostess Fruit Pie	1 pie	420	20.0	1.0
Lemon Chiffon, 1 Crust, Baked	1 cup	454	18.3	0.5
Lemon Meringue - Sara Lee	1/6 pie	350	5.0	5.0

ITEM NAME	PORTION	CAL	FAT	FIBER
Mince - Mrs. Smith's	⅙ pie	300	11.0	2.0
Peach - Hostess Fruit Pie	1 pie	400	18.0	2.0
Pecan, 1 Crust, Baked	1 cup	748	41.0	3.1
Pineapple - Hostess Fruit Pie	1 pie	400	16.0	2.0
Pumpkin, 1 Crust, Baked	1 cup	378	20.0	2.8
Pumpkin Custard - Mrs. Smith's	⅕ pie	270	8.0	1.0
Rhubarb, 2 Crusts, Baked	1 cup	486	20.5	3.1
Strawberry, 1 Crust, Baked	1 cup	345	13.7	3.7
Strawberry - Hostess Fruit Pie	1 pie	390	18.0	2.0
Sweet Potato, 1 Crust, Baked	1 cup	381	20.2	2.0
Pie Crust, Baked, Prepared from Mix	1 item	743	46.5	4.2
Pie Crust, Graham - Keebler	1 slice	110	5.0	0.4
Pie Filling, Cherry, Canned	1 serv.	85	0.2	0.5
Pie Filling, Apple, Canned	1 serv.	74	0.1	0.3

PUDDINGS

ITEM NAME	PORTION	CAL	FAT	FIBER
Chocolate				
Dry Mix - Jell-O	¼ pkg.	90	0.0	1.0
Rte* - Hunt's	1 serv.	160	6.0	0.0
Sugar-Free, Dry Mix - Jell-O	¼ pkg.	30	0.0	1.0
Chocolate Fudge, Lite, Rte - Jell-O	1 serv.	101	1.0	0.1
Chocolate/Caramel, Rte - Jell-O	1 serv.	175	6.0	0.8
Chocolate/Vanilla, Lite, Rte - Jell-O	1 serv.	104	2.0	0.8
Coconut, Instant	1 serv.	383	4.1	0.1
Coconut Cream, Regular - Dry	1 serv.	345	4.8	0.1
Corn	1 cup	273	13.3	1.1
Custard, Baked	1 cup	305	15.0	1.0
Double Chocolate - Yoplait	1 serv.	180	4.0	0.8
Flan, Caramel Custard, Prepared, 2% Milk	1 cup	270	4.6	0.9
Fudge/Milk Chocolate, Rte - Jell-O	1 serv.	171	6.0	0.8
Gelatin, Typical Variety with or w/o Sugar	1 oz.	18	0.0	0.0
Lemon, Dry Mix - Jell-O	⅙ pkg.	50	0.0	0.0
Milk Chocolate, Rte - Jell-O	1 serv.	173	6.0	0.1
Mousse, Chocolate, Instant, Prep - San Sucre	1 cup	150	3.0	0.0
Mousse - Home Recipe	1 cup	894	65.8	2.2
Rennin, Chocolate, Prepared with 2% Milk	1 cup	220	5.6	0.1

*Ready to eat.

ITEM NAME	PORTION	CAL	FAT	FIBER
Rice with Raisins	1 cup	387	8.2	1.4
Tapioca Cream, Starch - Home Recipe	1 cup	220	8.0	0.6
Vanilla, Regular, Dry	1 serv.	325	0.4	0.1
Vanilla/Chocolate, Rte - Jell-O	1 serv.	178	6.0	0.8
York Peppermint Patty - Hershey	1 item	180	6.0	0.8

OTHER PASTRIES & SWEETS

ITEM NAME	PORTION	CAL	FAT	FIBER
Apple Butter	1 tbsp.	37	0.2	0.2
Apple Crisp, Berkshire - Pepperidge	1 oz.	53	1.7	0.5
Apple Crisp, Easy Delicious - Betty Crocker	⅛ pkg.	310	11.0	3.0
Apple Dumplings - Pepperidge	1 oz.	87	4.3	0.4
Banana Chips	1 oz.	147	9.5	1.9
Carob Powder	1 oz.	51	0.4	2.0
Carob Chips	1 serv.	151	9.4	1.8
✔ Chutney, Mango Type	1 cup	632	0.1	6.9
Cobbler, Frozen - Weight Watchers	1 slice	160	6.0	0.9
Coconut Cream, Raw	1 cup	792	83.2	1.6
Coconut Milk, Raw	1 cup	552	57.2	1.1
Danish				
Black Forest, Fat Free - Entenmann's	⅛ piece	130	0.0	2.0
Orange with Icing - Pillsbury	1 item	150	7.0	0.6
Plain	1 item	250	13.6	0.6
Eclair, Custard with Chocolate Icing	1 item	239	13.6	0.5
Eclair, Weight Watchers	1 item	150	5.0	2.0
Grapefruit, Peel, Candied	1 cup	536	0.5	4.4
Honey, Strained/Extracted	1 tbsp.	65	0.0	0.1
Honey, Strained or Extracted	1 cup	1016	0.0	0.7
Jam/Preserves	1 cup	870	0.3	2.9
Regular	1 tbsp.	55	0.0	0.2
Strawberry, Low Calorie	1 tsp.	8	0.0	0.1
Lemon Peel, Candied	1 cup	670	0.6	5.5
✔ Marmalade, Citrus	1 cup	822	0.3	16.0
Marmalade (Marmalad)	1 oz.	67	0.1	0.1
Muffin, Apple Streusel - Hostess Breakfast	1 item	100	1.0	1.0
Muffin, Blueberry - Hostess Breakfast	1 item	100	1.0	1.0
✔ Orange Peel, Candied	1 cup	536	0.5	5.8
Pastry Pockets - Pillsbury	1 item	240	13.0	1.0
Pears, Candied	1 cup	566	1.1	3.7
Pecan Danish Ring - Entenmann's	⅛ piece	130	15.0	1.0
Pecan Spinners - Hostess	1 piece	110	5.0	0.8

ITEM NAME	PORTION	CAL	FAT	FIBER
Pineapple, Candied	1 cup	590	0.7	0.7
Raspberry Cheese, Fat Free - Entenmann's	1/8 piece	140	0.0	1.0
Roll, Cinnamon with Icing - Pillsbury	1 item	110	5.0	0.4
Rolls & Buns, Sweet Rolls, Ready to Serve	1 cup	356	10.2	2.1
Sugar, Beet, Maple or Cane	1 cup	666	0.0	0.9
Swirls, Caramel Pecan - Hostess	1 swirl	250	15.0	1.0
Toaster Pastries, Strawberry- Kellogg's Pop Tarts	1 item	210	6.0	1.0
Toaster Pastries, Frosted Blueberry/ Cherry - Kellogg's Pop Tarts	1 item	200	5.0	1.0
Topping, Strawberry or Pineapple	1 cup	863	0.5	2.4
Turnover				
Apple - Pepperidge	1 item	330	14.0	6.0
Apple - Pillsbury	1 item	170	8.0	0.9
Cherry - Pepperidge	1 item	320	13.0	6.0
Cherry - Pillsbury	1 item	170	8.0	0.7
Peach - Pepperidge	1 item	340	15.0	6.0
Twinkie - Hostess	2 items	280	9.0	0.8

VEGETABLES

Whether they are fresh, dried, or canned, the vegetable section is a great place to find fiber-rich foods. Top contributors are the legumes, which include all varieties of fresh and canned beans, lentils, and peas. Other vegetable standouts include artichokes, broccoli, brussels sprouts, cabbage, and cauliflower. But, as you'll see, virtually all vegetables contribute. By including at least 3 to 5 servings of vegetables per day you'll be taking a big step toward a healthful, high-fiber diet.

ITEM NAME	PORTION	CAL	FAT	FIBER
FRESH, FROZEN, & DRIED VEGETABLES				
Alfalfa Seeds, Sprouted, Raw	1 cup	10	0.2	0.7
Amaranth, Boiled, Drained	1 cup	28	0.2	12.5
Amaranth, Raw	1 cup	7	0.1	2.8
Artichoke, Edible from One Medium Sized	1 serv.	25	0.0	3.0

ITEM NAME	PORTION	CAL	FAT	FIBER
✔ Artichoke Hearts - Boiled	1 cup	84	0.6	8.3
Asparagus	5 spears	20	0.0	2.0
Frozen, Boiled, Drained, Tips	1 cup	50	0.8	2.2
Bamboo Shoots, Fresh	1 cup	41	0.5	3.9
Beans				
✔ Adzuki, Boiled	1 cup	294	0.2	14.3
✔ Baked Beans - Home Recipe	1 cup	382	13.0	19.5
✔ Black, Cooked, Boiled	1 cup	227	0.9	7.2
✔ Cranberry, Boiled	1 cup	240	0.8	9.8
✔ French, Cooked, Boiled	1 cup	228	1.3	14.9
✔ Great Northern, Cooked, Drained	1 cup	208	0.8	9.7
Green, Frozen, Boiled - Health Valley	1 cup	50	2.0	2.0
Green Snap, Fresh	1 cup	19	0.0	4.0
✔ Honey Baked/Organic - Health Valley	1 cup	220	0.0	14.0
Italian/Green/Yellow, Boiled	1 cup	44	0.4	3.0
Italian/Green/Yellow, Frozen, Boiled	1 cup	35	0.2	3.4
✔ Kidney, All Types, Boiled	1 cup	225	0.9	8.6
✔ Lima, Baby or Large, Boiled	1 cup	223	0.7	12.6
✔ Lima, Frozen, Boiled - Health Valley	1 cup	50	2.0	14.0
✔ Mung, Boiled	1 cup	213	0.8	10.6
Mung, Sprouted, Boiled	1 cup	26	0.1	2.7
Mung, Sprouted, Raw	1 cup	31	0.2	1.6
✔ Mung, Mature, Stir Fried	1 cup	62	0.3	6.4
✔ Navy, Boiled	1 cup	259	1.0	10.1
✔ Navy Pea, Dry, Cooked, Drained	1 cup	225	1.0	9.3
✔ Pink, Boiled	1 cup	252	0.8	8.2
✔ Pinto, Boiled	1 cup	235	0.9	12.7
✔ Refried	1 cup	271	2.7	11.6
✔ White, Boiled	1 cup	249	0.6	8.7
Winged, Boiled	1 cup	252	10.1	3.1
Yardlong, Boiled	1 cup	202	0.8	3.1
Yellow, Boiled	1 cup	254	1.9	2.2
Yellow Wax, Fresh	1 cup	19	0.0	4.0
✔ Beets, Boiled, Drained	1 cup	77	0.1	5.4
Beets, Fresh	1 med.	50	0.5	2.0
Beet Greens, Boiled, Drained	1 cup	39	0.3	4.4
Bell Pepper, Green	1 med.	30	0.2	2.4
Bell Pepper, Red	1 med.	35	0.0	4.0
Broccoli				
✔ Fresh, Boiled, Drained	1 cup	43	0.5	5.4
Fresh, Medium Size	1 stalk	50	0.5	4.0
Frozen, Boiled - Health Valley	1 cup	50	2.0	4.0

74

ITEM NAME	PORTION	CAL	FAT	FIBER
Brussels Sprouts				
Fresh	4 items	40	0.5	3.0
Fresh, Boiled	1 cup	61	0.8	6.7
Frozen, Boiled	1 cup	65	0.6	6.4
Cabbage				
Celery, Fresh	1 cup	12	0.2	0.8
Chinese, Fresh	1 cup	6	0.0	0.3
Green, Boiled, Drained	1 cup	31	0.4	4.0
Green, Fresh	1/12 med.	25	0.0	0.2
Red, Fresh, Shredded	1 cup	19	0.2	1.4
Savoy, Fresh, Shredded	1 cup	19	0.1	1.5
Swamp, Boiled, Drained	1 cup	20	0.2	2.7
White Mustard, Boiled	1 cup	20	0.3	2.7
White Mustard, Fresh	1 cup	9	0.1	0.7
Carrots				
Boiled, Drained, Sliced	1 cup	70	0.3	5.8
Fresh, Scraped	1 med.	40	0.1	3.0
Fresh, Scraped, Shredded	1 cup	47	0.2	3.5
Cauliflower, Fresh, Medium				
Head	1/6 head	25	0.0	2.4
Cauliflower, Frozen, Boiled	1 cup	34	0.4	3.2
Celery				
Boiled	1 cup	42	0.4	4.2
Fresh	1 stalk	13	0.0	1.0
Fresh, Diced	1 cup	19	0.2	1.9
Chard, Swiss, Boiled, Drained	1 cup	35	0.1	3.7
Chard, Swiss, Fresh	1 cup	7	0.0	0.6
Chayote, Fruit, Raw	1/2 fruit	28	0.1	0.7
Chicory Greens, Fresh, Chopped	1 cup	41	0.5	4.3
Chives, Freeze Dried	1 tbsp.	3	0.0	0.1
Chives, Fresh	1 tbsp.	3	0.0	0.1
Collards, Fresh, Boiled, Drained	1 cup	35	0.2	2.1
Collards, Frozen, Cooked	1 cup	60	0.8	2.0
Corn				
Frozen, Boiled, Health Valley	1 cup	160	2.0	4.0
Sweet, Fresh (Med. Size)	1 ear	75	1.0	1.0
Cowpeas, Common, Pods &				
Seeds, Cooked	1 cup	54	0.5	2.7
Cress, Garden, Boiled	1 cup	31	0.8	1.2
Cress, Garden, Fresh	1 cup	16	0.4	0.6
Cucumber, Fresh	1 cup	29	0.3	2.0
Cucumber, Fresh	1/3 med.	15	0.0	0.5
Dandelion Greens, Boiled	1 cup	35	0.6	4.1
Dandelion Greens, Fresh	1 cup	25	0.4	1.9
Dock, Boiled, Drained	1 cup	38	0.4	1.4
Dock, Fresh	1 cup	39	0.4	1.1

ITEM NAME	PORTION	CAL	FAT	FIBER
Eggplant				
Boiled, Drained	1 cup	27	0.2	2.0
Fresh, Med. Size	1/5 item	25	0.0	2.0
Fresh, Med. Size	1 cup	22	0.0	2.0
Endive, Fresh, Chopped	1 cup	13	0.0	1.3
Fennel, Leaves	1 cup	17	0.2	0.3
Garlic, Fresh, Clove	1 clove	5	0.0	0.0
Ginger Root, Fresh, Sliced	1 cup	66	0.7	0.7
Gourd, White Flowered, Boiled	1 cup	22	0.0	1.6
Grits, Hominy, Cooked	1 cup	123	0.2	0.2
Horseradish, Fresh	1 cup	206	0.7	4.7
Horseradish, Raw	1 tbsp.	13	0.0	0.4
Hyacinth Beans, Fresh Pods	1 cup	32	0.3	1.6
Jerusalem Artichokes, Fresh	1 cup	114	0.0	2.0
Kale, Fresh, Boiled, Drained	1 cup	42	0.5	4.3
Kale, Frozen, Boiled, Drained	1 cup	39	0.6	3.8
Kohlrabi, Boiled, Drained	1 cup	48	0.2	3.3
Kohlrabi, Fresh	1 cup	38	0.1	2.6
Lamb's Quarter, Boiled, Drained	1 cup	64	1.4	3.6
Lamb's Quarter, Fresh	1 cup	14	0.3	0.7
Leeks, Boiled, Drained	1 item	38	0.2	4.0
Leeks, Fresh	1 item	76	0.4	2.5
✔ Lentils, Sprouted, Fresh	1 cup	82	0.4	6.2
✔ Lentils, Whole, Cooked	1 cup	231	0.7	9.8
Lettuce				
Butterhead, Head	1 item	21	0.4	1.6
Butterhead, Leaves	1 slice	2	0.0	0.2
Iceberg, Fresh, Med. Head	1/6 item	20	0.0	1.0
Leaf, Fresh, Shredded	1 cup	13	0.0	0.8
Looseleaf, Fresh	1 cup	10	0.2	0.8
Romaine, Fresh, Shredded	1 cup	9	0.1	1.0
✔ Miso, Fermented Soybeans	1 cup	567	16.7	9.9
Mixed Vegetables, Frozen,				
Boiled - Health Valley	1 cup	140	2.0	4.0
Mushrooms				
Fresh	5 med.	20	0.0	0.0
Shiitake, Cooked	1 cup	80	0.3	3.1
Shiitake, Dried	1 item	11	0.0	0.4
Mustard Greens				
Boiled, Drained	1 cup	21	0.3	2.7
Fresh	1 cup	10	0.2	0.4
Frozen, Boiled	1 cup	28	0.4	2.9
Okra, Fresh	6 pods	30	0.0	1.0
Okra, Fresh, Boiled, Drained	1 cup	51	0.3	2.0
Onions				
Boiled	1 cup	98	0.4	3.8

ITEM NAME	PORTION	CAL	FAT	FIBER
Fresh, Med. Size	1 item	60	0.0	3.1
Green, Chopped	1 cup	40	0.0	3.0
Mature, Fresh, Chopped	1 cup	61	0.3	2.7
Parsley, Fresh, Chopped	1 cup	22	0.5	2.0
Parsnips, Fresh	1 large	132	1.0	4.0
Parsnips, Sliced, Boiled, Drained	1 cup	126	0.5	7.6
Peas				
Blackeye/Cowpeas, Boiled, Drained	1 cup	179	1.3	15.8
Blackeye/Cowpeas, Fresh, Boiled	1 cup	160	0.6	11.0
Blackeye/Cowpeas, Frozen, Boiled	1 cup	224	1.1	9.8
Edible Podded, Boiled	1 cup	67	0.4	4.2
Edible Podded, Fresh	1 cup	61	0.3	3.8
Green, Fresh	1 cup	117	0.6	4.9
Green, Fresh, Boiled	1 cup	134	0.3	5.4
Green, Frozen, Boiled - Health Valley	1 cup	160	2.0	6.0
Split, Boiled	1 cup	231	0.8	8.0
Split, Dry, Cooked	1 cup	230	1.0	10.5
Split, Fresh	1 cup	671	2.3	8.1
Peas & Carrots, Frozen, Boiled	1 cup	77	0.7	7.1
Peas & Onions, Frozen, Boiled	1 cup	81	0.4	4.7
Peppers				
Bell, Green, Red, Yellow, Fresh	1 med.	30	0.0	2.0
Hot, Red, Dried	1 tsp.	5	0.0	0.7
Hot Chili, Fresh	1 cup	60	0.3	3.6
Hot Chili, Red Pods with Seeds	1 med.	93	2.3	9.0
Jalapeno, Rosarita	1 item	7	0.0	0.4
Mexican, Hot, Tiny - Vlasic	1 oz.	6	0.0	0.4
Pickle				
Chowchow, Sour	1 cup	70	3.1	3.6
Chowchow, Sweet	1 cup	284	2.2	3.7
Crunchy Dills, Kosher - Vlasic	1 oz.	4	0.0	0.4
Cucumber, Fresh, Bread & Butter	1 cup	124	0.3	2.6
Cucumber, Dill	1 cup	28	0.3	1.7
Cucumber, Dill, Med. Sized	1 item	5	0.0	0.8
Cucumber, Dill, Whole, 3¾"	1 item	12	0.4	0.7
Dill, Low Sodium	1 item	12	0.1	1.0
Sweet/Gherkin, Small, Whole	1 item	20	0.0	0.2
Potato				
Fresh, Flesh	1 cup	190	0.2	3.6
Fresh, Flesh & Skin	1 cup	181	0.2	4.0
Fresh, Whole	1 med.	120	0.0	2.6
Baked, Flesh Only	1 cup	237	0.3	5.5
Baked, Flesh & Skin	1 cup	257	0.2	5.9

ITEM NAME	PORTION	CAL	FAT	FIBER
Baked, Skin Only, Med. Sized	1 item	115	0.1	3.0
✔ Baked in Microwave, Flesh/Skin	1 cup	237	0.2	5.6
French Fried, Restaurant				
Cooked	1 cup	180	6.0	2.4
Frozen, Fried in Oil	1 cup	180	9.4	2.0
Hash Brown, Prepared from				
Fresh	1 cup	239	21.7	3.1
Hash Brown, Prepared from				
Frozen	1 cup	340	17.9	1.5
Mashed, from Dehydrated,				
with Milk	1 cup	166	4.6	1.2
Mashed, from Fresh, with Milk	1 cup	162	1.2	1.2
Potato Puffs, Frozen, Heated	1 item	16	0.8	0.2
Prickly Pear, Fresh, Average Size	1 item	27	0.1	1.0
Prickly Pear, Fresh, with Seeds,				
Average Size	1 item	39	0.9	4.3
Pumpkin				
✔ Boiled, Drained, Mashed	1 cup	49	0.2	6.7
Canned	1 cup	80	0.7	3.2
Fresh, Cubed	1 cup	30	0.1	2.0
Purslane, Leaves & Stems,				
Boiled & Drained	1 cup	13	0.3	0.7
Purslane, Leaves & Stems, Raw	1 cup	13	0.2	0.5
Radish				
Daikon, Sliced, Boiled, Drained	1 cup	25	0.4	2.9
Oriental, Fresh	1 cup	18	0.1	0.7
Red, Fresh	1 item	2	0.0	0.1
Rutabagas				
Boiled, Drained, Cubes	1 cup	70	0.2	2.2
✔ Swedes, Boiled	1 cup	83	0.5	5.1
Swedes, Fresh	1 oz.	10	0.1	0.7
Salsify, Boiled, Drained	1 cup	62	0.9	2.7
Seaweed				
Dried (Hai-Tai)	1 oz.	71	0.3	2.1
Irishmoss, Fresh	1 oz.	14	0.0	1.0
Kelp (Kombu), Fresh	1 oz.	12	0.2	1.2
Laver (Nori), Fresh	1 oz.	10	0.1	1.0
Spirulina, Dried	1 oz.	82	2.2	1.4
Wakame, Fresh	1 oz.	13	0.2	1.2
Shallots, Fresh	3 tbsp.	20	0.0	0.2
Soybeans				
✔ Boiled	1 cup	298	15.4	7.5
✔ Dry Roasted	1 cup	775	37.2	7.5
✔ Roasted	1 cup	811	43.7	7.5
Sprouted, Boiled & Drained	1 cup	48	1.8	1.0
Sprouted, Fresh	1 cup	48	1.5	0.8

ITEM NAME	PORTION	CAL	FAT	FIBER
Spinach				
Fresh, Boiled, Drained	1 cup	41	0.5	4.0
Frozen, Boiled - Health Valley	1 cup	50	2.0	4.0
Raw	1 cup	27	0.0	3.3
Squash				
Acorn, Baked	1 cup	113	0.2	3.7
Butternut, Baked	1 cup	139	0.2	3.7
Crookneck, Fresh	1 cup	20	0.0	2.0
Hubbard, Baked	1 cup	103	0.8	3.7
Spaghetti, Fresh	1 cup	50	0.0	2.0
Zucchini, Boiled	1 cup	38	0.3	3.2
Zucchini, Fresh, Sliced	1 cup	18	0.2	1.2
Squash Flowers	1 large	3	0.1	0.1
Succotash (Corn & Lima Beans)	1 cup	150	0.6	1.4
Sweet Potato, Fresh	1 med.	140	0.0	3.0
Sweet Potato, Baked, Peeled	1 item	117	0.1	3.4
Taro Root (Poi)	1 cup	269	0.3	4.8
Tofu				
Fresh, Firm	1 cup	365	22.0	3.0
Fried	1 piece	35	2.6	0.2
Okara	1 cup	94	2.1	5.0
Soybean Curd, Fresh, Regular	1 piece	88	5.6	1.4
Tofu Silken				
Extra Firm, Mori Nu, 1" Slice	1 slice	90	3.2	0.0
Firm, Mori Nu, 1" Slice	1 slice	90	4.0	0.0
Soft, Mori Nu, 1" Slice	1 slice	80	4.2	0.0
Tomatillo, Fresh, Chopped	1 cup	42	1.4	2.6
Tomato				
Cooked, Stewed - Home Recipe	1 cup	80	2.7	1.0
Diced	1 cup	47	0.6	1.9
Diced, in Puree - Hunt's	1 serv.	24	0.2	2.3
Fresh	1 med.	35	0.0	1.0
Green, Fresh	1 small	24	0.2	0.5
Paste - Hunt's	1 serv.	92	0.4	4.3
Powder	1 oz.	86	0.1	0.7
Puree - Hunt's	1 serv.	52	0.2	2.3
Red, Fresh, Boiled	1 cup	65	1.0	2.4
Red, Ripe, Boiled	1 cup	62	0.5	1.4
Stewed - Hunt's	1 serv.	29	0.2	2.1
Turnips, Boiled, Drained	1 cup	35	0.3	1.4
Turnips, Fresh	1 cup	40	0.3	1.2
Turnip Greens, Boiled	1 cup	29	0.3	4.5
Turnip Greens, Fresh	1 cup	56	0.6	1.6
Waterchestnuts, Fresh	1 cup	57	0.1	0.7
Watercress, Leaves & Stems, Fresh	1 cup	7	0.1	0.2
Yambean, Raw, Cubed	1 cup	77	0.3	1.0

ITEM NAME	PORTION	CAL	FAT	FIBER
Yams, Boiled or Baked, Drained	1 cup	158	0.2	3.3

CANNED

ITEM NAME	PORTION	CAL	FAT	FIBER
Artichoke Hearts, Marinated, Quartered - S&W	2 pieces	20	2.0	1.0
Asparagus				
Blended - S&W	6 pieces	15	0.0	1.0
Dietary Pack, Low Sodium	1 cup	34	0.5	3.9
Spears, Drained	1 cup	46	1.6	3.9
Bamboo Shoots - La Choy	1 cup	25	0.5	2.0
Beans				
✔ Adzuki, Sweetened	1 cup	702	0.1	13.7
✔ Baked Beans	1 cup	236	1.1	19.6
✔ Baked with Pork	1 cup	268	3.9	13.9
✔ Black - Sun-Vista	1 cup	140	2.0	14.0
✔ Black - S&W	1 cup	140	0.0	12.0
✔ Black Eye - Sun Vista	1 cup	140	0.0	8.0
Boston Baked, Fat Free - Health Valley	1 oz.	25	0.1	0.7
✔ Brick Oven Baked - S&W	1 cup	320	1.0	14.0
✔ Butter - S&W	1 cup	140	0.0	10.0
✔ Chili - Sun Vista	1 cup	220	2.0	14.0
✔ Garbanzo - S&W	1 cup	160	3.0	14.0
✔ Great Northern - Sun Vista	1 cup	140	0.0	12.0
Green, Dietary, Low Sodium	1 cup	26	0.1	2.6
Green - S&W	1 cup	40	0.0	4.0
Green & Wax - S&W	1 cup	40	0.0	4.0
Homestyle - Campbell's	1 oz.	28	0.5	1.6
✔ Honey Baked, Fat Free - Health Valley	1 cup	110	0.0	7.0
✔ Hot Chipotle Chili - S&W	1 cup	180	0.0	12.0
Hot Chili - Campbell's	1 oz.	23	0.5	0.4
✔ Hot Chili - Luck's	1 cup	240	2.0	12.0
Italian/Green/Yellow	1 cup	27	0.1	2.9
✔ Kidney, All Types	1 cup	207	0.8	13.3
✔ Kidney, Dietary, Low Sodium	1 cup	230	1.0	12.5
✔ Kidney, Light Red - Luck's	1 cup	240	0.0	10.0
✔ Kidney, Special Cook - Luck's	1 cup	220	0.0	14.0
✔ Lima, Solids & Liquids	1 cup	186	0.7	10.4
✔ Lima, Dietary, Low Sodium	1 cup	186	0.7	10.4
✔ Pinquitos - S&W	1 cup	160	1.0	12.0
✔ Pinto, Texas Style Barbecue - S&W	1 cup	200	3.0	16.0
✔ Pinto - Sun-Vista	1 cup	160	1.0	6.0
✔ Pinto, Smokey Ranch Beans - S&W	1 cup	220	5.0	12.0

ITEM NAME	PORTION	CAL	FAT	FIBER
Red, Cajun Style Beans - S&W	1 cup	160	4.0	16.0
Red Kidney, Solids & Liquids	1 cup	230	0.9	12.5
Refried, Sausage - Old El Paso	1 cup	388	26.0	6.0
Refried, Vegetarian or Spicy - Rosarita	1 cup	240	5.0	14.0
Shelling	1 cup	74	0.5	12.0
Snap, Green, Drained, Cuts	1 cup	27	0.1	1.8
Snap, with Liquids	1 cup	36	0.2	3.0
Snap, Yellow/Wax	1 cup	27	0.1	1.8
Vegetarian - Heinz	1 cup	130	1.0	7.0
Wax - S&W	1 cup	40	0.0	2.0
White, Small, Maple Sugar - S&W	1 cup	300	1.0	12.0
Bean Salad, Deli Style - S&W	1 cup	160	0.0	8.0
Bean Salad, Marinated - S&W	1 cup	140	0.0	6.0
Bean Sprouts - La Choy	1 cup	11	0.2	1.3
Beets				
Dietary Pack, Low Sodium	1 cup	71	0.2	4.2
Drained Solids	1 cup	77	0.3	4.2
Pickled, with Liquids	1 cup	149	0.2	3.4
Sliced, Drained	1 cup	53	0.2	2.9
Sliced - S&W	1 cup	60	0.0	2.0
Solids/Liquid	1 cup	84	0.2	1.2
Whole	1 cup	71	0.2	2.7
Carrots				
Dietary Pack, Low Sodium	1 cup	57	0.4	2.7
Sliced, Drained	1 cup	34	0.3	2.2
Sliced - S&W	1 cup	50	1.0	4.0
Chestnuts, Water - La Choy	1 cup	75	0.2	3.3
Chop Suey Vegetables - La Choy	1 cup	17	0.1	0.0
Corn				
Cream Style	1 cup	184	1.1	3.3
Cream Style - S&W	1 cup	200	2.0	2.0
Drained	1 cup	134	1.7	3.1
Frozen, Boiled, Drained	1 cup	134	0.1	3.5
Low Sodium	1 cup	156	1.2	4.9
Vacuum Pack, Niblets	1 cup	166	1.1	4.3
Whole Kernel - S&W	1 cup	180	2.0	4.0
with Red and Green Peppers	1 cup	170	1.3	5.1
Cowpeas, Common, Canned, with Pork	1 cup	199	3.8	15.4
Garden Salad, Dill - S&W	1 cup	100	0.0	6.0
Garden Salad, Marinated - S&W	1 cup	100	0.0	6.0
Hominy, White or Golden - Van Camp's	1 cup	160	2.0	2.0

ITEM NAME	PORTION	CAL	FAT	FIBER
Mixed Chinese Vegetables -				
La Choy	1 cup	17	0.1	0.3
Mixed Vegetables - S&W	1 cup	70	0.0	4.0
Mushrooms, Drained	1 item	3	0.0	0.3
✔ Mushrooms, Drained Solids	1 cup	61	0.7	6.4
Olives				
Green, Pickled	1 item	4	0.5	0.1
Mission, Ripe	1 item	5	0.7	0.1
✔ Pickled/Canned or Bottled,				
Green	1 item	171	18.7	6.5
Onions, Solids and Liquids	1 cup	22	0.3	3.0
Peas				
✔ Green	1 cup	117	0.6	7.7
✔ Green, Dietary, Low Sodium	1 cup	117	0.6	5.8
✔ Green - Sun Vista	1 cup	160	0.0	10.0
✔ Green - S&W	1 cup	140	0.0	8.0
✔ Petit Pois - S&W	1 cup	140	0.0	8.0
✔ Peas & Carrots	1 cup	97	0.7	8.6
✔ S&W	1 cup	100	0.0	6.0
✔ Dietary, Low Sodium	1 cup	96	0.7	7.1
Peas & Onions	1 cup	61	0.5	4.3
✔ S&W	1 cup	80	0.0	6.0
Peppers, Hot Chili	1 cup	34	0.1	2.1
Peppers, Jalapeno, Chopped	1 cup	33	0.8	2.0
Pimento, Med. Sized	1 med.	11	0.2	0.2
Potatoes, Solids & Liquid	1 cup	110	0.5	0.5
Potatoes, New - S&W	1 cup	120	0.0	2.0
✔ Pumpkin	1 cup	83	0.7	7.1
✔ Pumpkin - Libby's	1 cup	80	1.0	10.0
Pumpkin Pie Mix - Libby's	1 cup	200	0.0	4.0
Sauerkraut, Solids & Liquid	1 cup	27	0.3	1.1
Spinach				
✔ Dietary Pack, Low Sodium	1 cup	45	0.9	5.1
✔ Drained	1 cup	50	1.1	6.8
✔ Solids and Liquids	1 cup	45	0.9	5.1
S&W	1 cup	60	0.0	4.0
Squash, Zucchini, Italian Style -				
Del Monte	1 cup	60	0.0	2.0
Succotash - S&W	1 cup	200	2.0	4.0
Sweet Potato				
Canned in Syrup, Drained	1 cup	213	0.6	3.3
Mashed	1 cup	258	0.5	4.6
Vacuum Pack	1 cup	182	0.4	4.8
Tomato, Red				
Dietary Pack, Low Sodium	1 cup	48	0.6	1.7
with Green Chilies	1 cup	36	0.2	0.9

ITEM NAME	PORTION	CAL	FAT	FIBER
Ripe, Stewed	1 cup	66	0.4	2.7
Ripe, Whole	1 cup	48	0.6	2.5
Stewed	1 cup	66	0.4	2.0
Stewed, Italian Recipe - S&W	1 cup	70	0.0	4.0
Whole	1 cup	48	0.6	1.7
Tomato Paste	1 cup	204	1.0	2.2
Low Sodium	1 cup	220	2.3	11.3
Salt Added	1 cup	220	2.3	11.3
Tomato Puree, Low Sodium	1 cup	103	0.3	5.8
Tomato Puree, Salt Added	1 cup	103	0.3	5.8
Waterchestnuts	1 cup	70	0.1	3.6
Yams, Old-Fashioned Candied - S&W	1 cup	340	0.0	8.0

MIXES ADDED TO VEGETABLES

ITEM NAME	PORTION	CAL	FAT	FIBER
Potatoes				
Homestyle, Broccoli Au Gratin	1 item	180	2.0	0.5
Homestyle, Cheesy Scalloped	1 item	180	2.0	0.5
Specialty, Au Gratin and Cheddar 'n Bacon, prepared - Betty Crocker	½ cup	100	1.5	1.0
Specialty, Hash Brown, prep. - Betty Crocker	½ cup	130	0.0	2.0
Specialty, Julienne - Betty Crocker	½ cup	90	1.0	1.0
Specialty, Scalloped - Betty Crocker	½ cup	100	1.5	1.0
Twice Baked, Bacon/Cheddar	⅔ cup	110	2.5	1.0
Twice Baked, Sour Cream/Chive	1 item	180	4.0	0.5
Potato Buds				
Betty Crocker	⅓ cup	80	0.5	1.0
Cheddar Cheese - Betty Crocker	⅓ cup	120	3.0	1.0
Sour Cream 'n Chive - Betty Crocker	⅓ cup	120	3.5	1.0
Potatoes Express				
Alfredo - Betty Crocker	⅔ cup	110	1.5	1.0
Broccoli Au Gratin - Betty Crocker	⅔ cup	100	1.0	1.0
Cheddar Cheese - Betty Crocker	⅔ cup	100	1.0	1.0
Creamy Scalloped - Betty Crocker	⅔ cup	110	2.0	1.0
Sour Cream/Chives - Betty Crocker	⅔ cup	110	1.5	1.0
Salad, Classic Pasta - Suddenly Salad	1 item	240	2.0	0.6
Salad, Pasta Primavera - Suddenly Salad	1 item	180	2.0	0.4